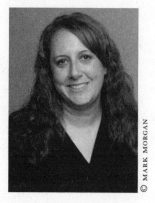

© MARK MORGAN

About the Author

HEATHER LAUER is a lifelong bacon enthusiast and the creator of the popular Web site BaconUnwrapped.com. She lives in Phoenix, Arizona and Fairfield, Idaho.

BACON: A LOVE STORY

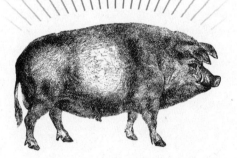

HEATHER LAUER

Packaged by Dolphin & Jones Book Packaging

WILLIAM MORROW

An Imprint of HarperCollins*Publishers*

THIS BOOK IS DEDICATED TO THE MIGHTY SWINE. WITHOUT THAT MAGNIFICENT BEAST, NONE OF US WOULD KNOW THE IMMENSE AND INFINITE PLEASURE THAT IS BACON. WE ARE NOT WORTHY.

Grateful acknowledgment is made to reprint the excerpt on page 51 from THE SIMPSONS TM and © 1998 Twentieth Century Fox Television. Written by David X. Cohen. All rights reserved.

A hardcover edition of this book was published in 2009 by William Morrow, an imprint of HarperCollins Publishers.

HarperCollins books may be purchased for educational, business, or sales promotional use. For information please write: Special Markets Department, HarperCollins Publishers, 10 East 53rd Street, New York, NY 10022.

FIRST HARPER PAPERBACK EDITION PUBLISHED 2010.

Designed by Allison Meierding
Original concept by Jessica Dorfman Jones
Developmental editor: Jessica Dorfman Jones

Library of Congress Cataloging-in-Publication Data
    Lauer, Heather.
        Bacon : a love story : a salty survey of everybody's favorite meat / Heather Lauer.
    —1st ed.
        p. cm.
    ISBN 978-0-06-170428-4
    1. Cookery (Bacon). 2. Bacon I. Title.
    TX749.5.P67L387 2009
    641.6'64—dc22   2009009691

ISBN 978-0-06-197126-6 (pbk.)

11 12 13 14 OV/RRD 10 9 8 7 6 5 4

Acknowledgments

I have several people to thank for my bacon education over the years, including some who are much smarter than I, and probably even more obsessed, when it comes to the wonderful world of bacon.

First of all, I must obviously thank my parents for allowing bacon to be a part of my childhood. We actually didn't eat it very often when I was growing up—it was normally reserved for holiday breakfasts or other special occasions—but clearly that first "taste" was enough to lead me to this point in my life. My parents also introduced me to beef bacon, another gustatory delight I indulge in with great pleasure. While not bacon in the truest sense, beef bacon is equally delicious and deserves to be served side by side with pork bacon in almost any setting.

My two brothers, Micah and Erich, also deserve some credit, because the idea for *Bacon Unwrapped* was actually born out of a spirited evening of cocktails and heated debate (aka an average Saturday night for us) that somehow led to an intense discussion about bacon being not only the Best Meat Ever but possibly the Best Food Ever. And within one week of that episode, my blog was launched. By the way, the marriage of booze and bacon is a theme I explore several times throughout this book—the two are connected in more ways than you might realize!

Of all the chefs, curers, farmers, and fanatics I interviewed for this book, there is one person who stands out as deserving special thanks. Chef Greggory Hill, formerly of the restaurant David Greggory in Washington, DC, is a fan of bacon like no other. In later chapters I'll tell you all about Chef Hill and the bacon-blessed menus he created and events he hosted at his restaurant. He graciously shared his knowledge and recipes with me on several occasions, and was an early supporter of this project.

One of the best things about writing this book has been all of the amazing members of the Bacon Nation I've had the honor of meeting, particularly those who hosted me during my cross-country "Bacon Tour of America" in 2008. Many of them were strangers to me before agreeing to be interviewed, but every single one of them was willing to take as much time as necessary to talk about the Best Meat Ever. The Bacon Nation is filled with many warm, caring people who are devoted to their beloved meat and are more than happy to share their experiences. So "thanks" to the following people for helping to make this book happen: Steve Wesley; David Lebovitz; Todd Kruse; Eric Savage; Brooks Reynolds; Herb Eckhouse of La Quercia; Ronny and Beth Drennan of Broadbent Hams; Jason Baskin of Hormel Foods; Leslie and June Scott; Nancy Newsom Mahaffey; Mike Sloan of Swiss Meats; Andy Thielen; Stefano Frigerio of Mio Restaurant in Washington, DC; Chef Todd Gray of Equinox in Washington, DC; Chef Ethan McKee of Rock Creek in Washington, DC; Chef Dustan Bristol of Brick 29 in Nampa, Idaho; Jeff Bruning of the High Life Lounge in Des Moines, Iowa; Chef Nathan Anda of Tallula in Arlington, Virginia; Sean Brock of McCrady's Restaurant in Charleston, South Carolina; Jason Lewis of Lollyphile; Cat Daddy, owner of Voodoo Doughnuts in Portland, Oregon; Brenda Beaman of Williamson Kenwood; and Rocco Loosbrock of Coastal Vineyards.

Many excellent pork-themed books have been written over the years, but two of my favorites that provided inspiration for my own effort are Bruce Aidell's *Complete Book of Pork* and Peter Kaminsky's *Pig Perfect: Encounters with Remarkable Swine and Some Great Ways to Cook Them*. These two books are a must-read for any true pork-lover.

I must also give a big thank-you to my editor at William Morrow, Anne Cole, as well as Jessica Jones and Laurie Dolphin at D&J Book Packaging and Media. As a first-time author, their support and guidance throughout the entire process of writing this book has been invaluable.

Last but not least, thanks to all my friends who have sampled my bacon desserts, attended bacon-themed dinners with me, e-mailed me their stories about bacon, given me bacon-themed gifts, and otherwise indulged my obsession during this unusual and unexpected journey. You're all troupers and hopefully you've had as much fun as I have!

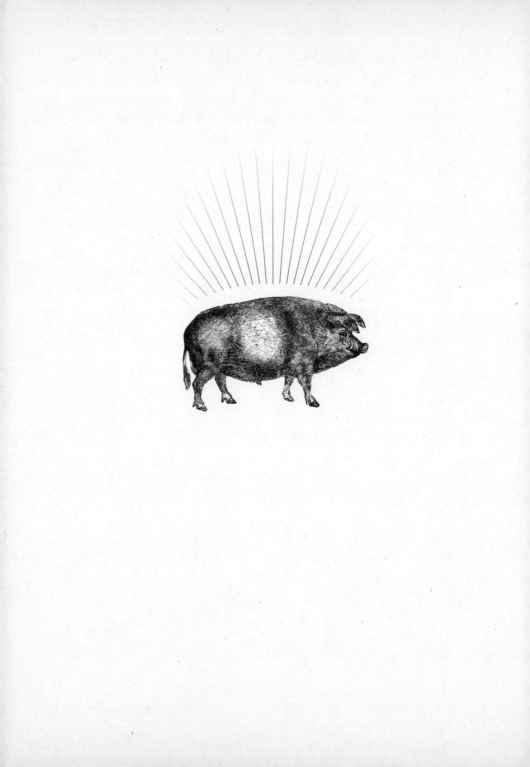

CONTENTS

Introduction

I bet you've eaten bacon in the last forty-eight hours.

Whether you purchased this book yourself, or someone saw it and thought of you, you are probably one of millions of Americans who have a condition called Obsession With Bacon (OWB). Otherwise it seems unlikely that you would be in possession of a literary work singularly focused on the Best Meat Ever (and yes, of course, I'm talking about bacon).

One of the symptoms of OWB is the need to find as many ways as possible to incorporate bacon into your daily diet. For some of you, this may be as simple as enjoying a strip (or ten) of bacon for breakfast every morning. For others it could mean a lunchtime BLT at your favorite neighborhood café. The über-obsessed might experiment with bacon in a dessert or cocktail. Regardless of the impact OWB has on your life, the common indicator for all sufferers of this condition is you've often got bacon on your mind.

I know because I, too, suffer from OWB.

I've got OWB so bad that one day during the summer of 2005, I decided to embark on a mission to learn as much as possible about the brilliant meat product that is bacon, and to share my passion with the world. And thus began my love affair with the Best Meat Ever that is *Bacon Unwrapped* (www.baconunwrapped.com).

The evolution of *Bacon Unwrapped*, and ultimately the process of writing this book, have led me to consume more bacon in the last couple of years than I ever would have imagined to be humanly possible. Now my friends and family automatically think of me every time they eat bacon, and there's nothing weirder than receiving an e-mail or call from someone who feels compelled to report that they had bacon for breakfast. I spend more time than is normal talking with perfect strangers about the best way to cook bacon. Friends regularly ask me to recommend a good brand of bacon. People buy me bacon-related gifts for my birthday and holidays—I've received the same "bacon wallet" from three different people, and I've got enough containers of "bacon band-aids" to take care of my cuts and scratches for the next couple of decades.

So suffice it to say, when I decided to launch *Bacon Unwrapped* on a whim that one summer afternoon, it changed my life in a very strange and unexpected way. What was once an occasional pleasure has evolved into an integral part of my daily existence on many different levels.

Bacon has also evolved over time, and it has come a long way from the days when it was cured mostly for practical reasons as a means of food preservation. What was once a survival tactic is now a passion for many people. These days bacon is available in a variety of flavors, and consumers have more options available to them than ever before. Some people are satisfied with the choices at their local supermarket. Others will travel long distances or pay shipping fees to acquire their favorite bacon, like groupies following their favorite rock band on a cross-country tour. Several companies are building a name for themselves as purveyors of specialty bacons, and the popularity of artisanal bacons is increasing exponentially as more and more people are exposed to these flavorful and unique products. These dealers in bacon are openly exploiting the needs of the most obsessed bacon addicts . . . and our palates are grateful.

Americans consumed 737 million pounds of bacon in 2006, according to the National Pork Board, equal to $2 billion worth of bacon. Bacon sales rose 20 percent from 2000 to 2005, a result of added flavors such as maple and jalapeño and the increased use of bacon to accompany other foods, according to the National Pork Board. Not only are we addicted to bacon but our addiction is growing more intense by the day. Fifty-three percent of households report having bacon on hand at all times. Having bacon in your home is just about as common as having basic household items such as laundry detergent and lightbulbs.

But the increase in bacon sales over the last several years is attributed more to restaurants than the individual consumer. Sixty-two percent of restaurants now have bacon on their menu, as more have included it in non-breakfast items such as sandwiches, pizzas, and salads, according to the Foodservice Research Institute. When Americans go out to eat, they are demanding more bacon . . . more bacon now! Chefs at restaurants around the United States are waking up to the fact that Americans just can't get enough of their darling meat, and bacon is increasingly appearing on menus ranging from your local greasy spoon to some of the top restaurants in the country. Baconmania has swept the country—join the movement or get out of the way!

To further prove the omnipresence of bacon, even the Internet is feeling the pressure of the bacon movement. A recent Google search for "bacon" yielded over 50 million results. Setting aside the pings related to Francis Bacon, Kevin Bacon, and all of the other individuals and locations that are lucky enough to have such a splendid name, the results include numerous Web sites where you can purchase specialty bacon, information about cooking bacon, countless recipes that feature bacon, blogs about bacon, a wide variety of bacon-inspired products ranging from bacon scarves to bacon scented candles, videos of people cooking and eating bacon, bacon-related humor, and chat rooms where people talk about nothing but their love of bacon. There are a lot of people in this world who are obsessed with bacon and aren't afraid to express themselves and their undying passion for cured pork belly. For these intrepid souls, bacon is clearly a source of joy, creativity, and daily inspiration. But for most, bacon is just a really delicious meat that appeals to our carnivorous instincts and attraction to foods that combine sweet and salty flavors. Bacon has been around for eons, and thanks to its greasy allure its popularity shows no signs of waning. And, oh yeah, bacon is simply the BEST MEAT EVER.

Bacon has been a source of amusement, some incredible meals, and even a few new friendships for me during the last couple of years. With this book, I share some of those meals and experiences with you, along with the knowledge I've collected along the way. Included are interviews with people I've met whose lives are impacted by bacon on a daily basis—the true Bacon Nation. This book is an exploration of bacon as food, culture, humor, adventure, and something that unifies humans on a very basic and primal level. While you may learn something from this book, I hope more than anything that you just have fun with it in the same way I've thoroughly enjoyed becoming a "bacon connoisseur." I also encourage you to try some of the recipes—particularly the quirkier ones. So go on, celebrate your Obsession With Bacon, and in the immortal words of Homer Simpson, "bacon up!"

PART I

BACON 101

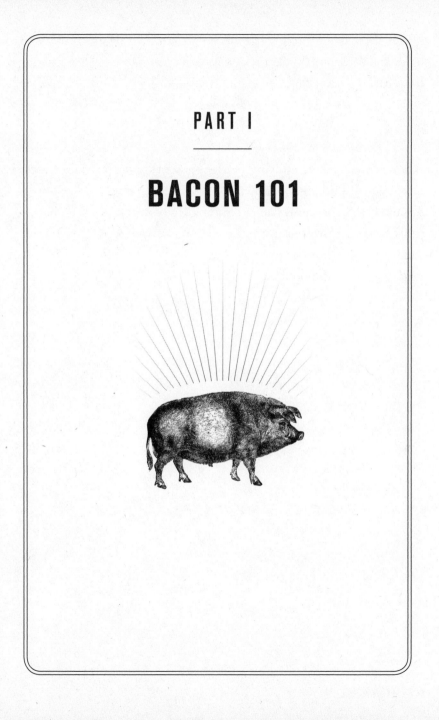

CHAPTER 1

ON THE EIGHTH DAY, GOD CREATED BACON

"Whenever I'm at a brunch buffet and they have that big
metal tray filled with the 4,000 pieces of bacon, I always
think, 'If I was here by myself . . . I would eat only bacon. I
would steal this tray, go lay down, and eat bacon all day.'"
—COMEDIAN JIM GAFFIGAN

MOST OF US take for granted that bacon can be readily purchased from grocery stores and butchers all over the world. Or that it can always be found in abundance at your neighborhood Eat-O-Rama (our love of trough-like eating is yet one of the many things humans and pigs have in common). But our good fortune regarding the widespread availability of bacon has been a long time coming. To understand why bacon is The Best Meat Ever, it's important to understand how it came to be a part of the human diet in the first place.

And make no mistake; bacon *is* absolutely The Best Meat Ever.

Humans have been consuming pork for thousands of years. While we may think of bacon as being inextricably linked to modern favorites like the bacon cheeseburger or BLT, it was a huge hit in the ancient world, too. It has been estimated that the first pig-like creatures were roaming the earth up to 40 million years ago in Asia and Europe, and eventually our ancestors figured out that these portly beasts could be a delicious form of sustenance. The Chinese got wise to the pleasures of pork early on and domesticated pigs by 4300 B.C. This probably was not a very difficult process—the pigs were likely to stick around simply if provided with a source of food (this is another thing pigs have in common with most humans, particularly those likely to be found attached to an all-you-can-eat buffet). Europeans got in on the act a little later and were enjoying bacon, chops, and the rest of the hog by 1500 B.C. And from that point on, the humble pig accompanied humans on their journeys around the globe.

Domesticated pigs were so popular during the Middle Ages that they wandered free through the streets of Europe. This wasn't an entirely bad thing, as the pigs helped with rubbish control, but it was also problematic because those peripatetic porkers often hung out in parts of the city where they weren't so welcome. In 1131, Prince Philip, son of Louis VI of France, was killed when his horse threw him after being startled by a stray pig. As a result, an attempt was made to pass a law forbidding the raising of pigs in town. But given the popularity of having instant access to delicious pork products, the law was largely ignored for several centuries.

Roving pigs weren't just a problem for European cities. Fast forward to colonial New York City where there was also a swine problem, as pigs would often run amok through farmers' grain fields. In an effort to keep the unruly hogs at bay, the residents of Manhattan erected a wall along the northern edge of the settlement. And the street that eventually bordered the wall was called Wall Street. Now that this area of New York City is overrun with stockbrokers and hedge fund managers, some might say the swine problem was never really solved.

Americans believe that we have Christopher Columbus and Hernando de Soto to thank for all the bacon, ribs, and tenderloins we enjoy, as they had pigs with them on their ships. Back when it took multiple weeks to cross the Atlantic Ocean on a journey to the New World, pigs were a popular travel companion (nowadays, not so much—unfortunately most airlines won't let you carry a pig on the plane even if it's small enough to fit underneath the seat in front of you, and U.S. Customs isn't so keen on the idea, either). Hogs were on board the Nina, Pinta, and Santa Maria, both as charming companions and good eats. Pigs were ideal animals to take on a voyage to the New World as they will eat pretty much anything, which makes them extremely easy to care for. They also reproduce rapidly, which made them a constantly reliable (not to mention constantly delectable) source of food when the explorers reached their destination.

When Columbus and de Soto arrived in the Americas, the pigs on board made a break for it, right along with the sailors. So Columbus's porkers were the first visitors to the Americas when he arrived at the mainland of South America in 1498 to explore the Orinoco River; de Soto's contribution to the pig population took place a few decades later in what is now Florida. Not surprisingly, Native Americans quickly became quite enamored with the appetizing meat these pigs provided. In fact, they liked it so much that they attacked members of de Soto's expedition to swipe some hogs. It is rumored that descendants of de Soto's pigs still roam wild in the South, so if you should run into one, take a moment to recognize that you are experiencing a real brush with history. Pigs continued to accompany immigrants to the United States over the next several centuries, and thanks to the immigrants' diverse backgrounds, the initial swine population was equally diverse and varied by region.

Florida is not the only place where battles reportedly broke out between settlers and Native Americans over the presence of pigs. The Camas Prairie of central Idaho was the site of struggles between the Bannock and Shoshone tribes and white settlers along the Oregon Trail in the 1800s. The prairie had been an important food source for natives for many generations because of the abundance of camas and yumpa plants, wildlife, and other food supplies. Apparently the settlers' pigs agreed that the prairie plants were a tasty treat. Upon arrival on the prairie, the hungry pigs proceeded to decimate the landscape by digging up and munching down on the camas bulbs. This wild behavior led to the start of the Bannock War. So while pigs might be a palatable source of bacon, chops, and hams, they can also be a major source of trouble!

As the midwestern United States emerged as a major region for corn and grain farming in the mid-1800s, it naturally also became a place to establish large hog farms due to the availability of feed at an affordable price. Refrigerated rail transportation was also introduced shortly after the end of the Civil War, making it possible to slaughter pigs closer to the point of production than the point of consumption, and allowing the shipment of pork products to consumers nationwide. Iowa, Illinois, Minnesota, Nebraska, Indiana, and Missouri quickly became the top hog producing states in the country. During this period, pork production increased exponentially. Iowa is still the top pork producing state in the United States, and most of our pork continues to come from this handful of midwestern states known as the "Hog Belt" (a term that could also be used to describe a fashion accessory, albeit one that sounds astonishingly unflattering).

Outside of the Hog Belt, North Carolina has established itself as a leading pork producing state in recent years, thanks to major technological improvements in the pork industry. By raising pigs with improved genetics resulting in higher reproductive rates and leaner meat and requiring less feed per pound, North Carolina hog farmers have been able to establish themselves as industry leaders. These methods have now been widely adopted in the industry everywhere else in the United States. As the second-largest pork producing state in the country, North Carolina has seen hogs surpass tobacco in revenue production. The countless barbecue joints on country roadsides and in every town of any size in North Carolina attest to this development and ensure that Carolinians are able to personally reap the benefits of their growing industry.

THE POWER OF PORK

We humans have long been addicted to sweet, juicy hams, succulent pork tenderloin, and, of course, the seductive taste of salty, smoky bacon. European peasants in the Middle Ages were particularly fond of pork, and getting their hands on a pork belly was a pretty special event. Such was the power of pork, so strong a symbol of affluence, that bacon would be hung from the rafters for all to see when visitors came to call. It was a sign of wealth that a man could "bring home the bacon," then and now.

Speaking of bringing home the bacon, no one knows for sure where the saying comes from. What we do know is that the first recorded use of the phrase took place in 1906 in Reno, Nevada (quite a far cry from European peasantry!). The story goes that Joe Gans, the first African-American boxer to win a world title, fought in a match with the formidable Oscar "Battling" Nelson in Nevada. Joe was the favorite in this championship fight for the lightweight title, and the Reno *Evening Gazette* reported on the event by tugging at readers' heartstrings. The following telegram Gans received from his mother was read by announcer Larry Sullivan:

"Joe, the eyes of the world are on you. Everybody says you ought to win. Peter Jackson will tell me the news and you bring back the bacon." (September 3, 1906)

After winning the title, Joe allegedly sent a telegram back to his mother stating simply, "Bringing home the bacon." No doubt mom was proud.

Another idiomatic gem that attests to the bona fides of bacon was born in the European feudal era. The story goes that lucky peasants who had enough bacon in the house to spare would cut off a little to share with guests in order to sit around and "chew the fat." While this is the commonly accepted origin for this beloved phrase, some believe that it comes from the Eskimo culture in which whale blubber was chewed—much like chewing gum—while relaxing and carrying on conversations. A slightly different take on the phrase is that it is the origin for the word "chat"—a natural blending of the words "chew" and "fat." We have Cockney slang to thank for that one; interestingly, it seems to be one of the only terms from this form of the English language that has been adopted in the United States. Once again, proof of the power of pork.

Our beloved porker's contribution doesn't end with clever phrases, bacon, or other savory treats. Lard was, until recently, another highly prized by-product, commonly used for cooking in the United States prior to World War II. During the war, pigs played a key role in defending our freedom, as most lard was diverted to the military for use in manufacturing explosives. Forced to find an alternative, Americans were urged to use vegetable oil instead for cooking. By the time the war was over, the American palate had adjusted to the blander (if healthier) option, and lard never made a widespread comeback thereafter (a tragedy for American taste buds).

Since the war, the U.S. pork industry has seen explosive growth, with most operations being consolidated into large-scale farms. In recent years there has been some controversy surrounding a few of these farms, as questions have been raised about their methods. But the fact is that most Americans today satisfy their pork cravings with meat from large-scale operations. In the 1950s there were nearly 3 million pork producers. Today there are approximately 67,000 producers, with 53 percent of farms raising 5,000 or more pigs per year, producing more than 2 billion pounds of bacon each year in the United States alone. The U.S. pork industry is the second largest in the world, tied with Denmark behind Canada.

Traditionally the most common swine breeds raised on American farms were Yorkshire, Berkshire, Hampshire, Chester White, Poland China, Duroc, Spotted, and Landrace. But in recent years, companies specializing in swine genetics have merged the best of the top breeds to create hybrid pigs for large-scale producers. The result: Super Pig. These Super Pigs are less prone to disease, produce more pigs per litter, and result in a more consistent product to deliver to consumers. Perhaps someday they will also be able to leap tall buildings in a single bound . . . or maybe even fly. Hybrid pigs also produce the leaner meat that most American consumers demand. So while most of these hybrids can trace their roots back to the breeds traditionally raised on farms in the United States, they are genetically modified versions of these breeds. While less common than the hybrid variety produced for mass-market consumption, Berkshire hogs are becoming increasingly popular with smaller-scale niche producers, as they have an elongated, lean body that is considered perfect for producing those long, tasty strips of cured pork belly goodness so many of us covet.

HOME ON THE RANGE (OR IN A BARN)

The natural instinct of a wild pig is to scavenge for food in fields and forests, their natural habitat. Pigs love to forage and dig for roots, nuts, and fruit. Nonetheless, wild pigs and domesticated pigs alike will eat almost anything, including household waste—a fact that, combined with their predisposition toward spending their days lounging in mud (pigs don't have sweat glands and need water or mud to cool off), fuels their reputation as "filthy" animals. Contrary to this popular belief, pigs are actually quite clean when they aren't covered in mud—for instance, they instinctually keep their eating and defecating areas separate when given ample space to live. So are pigs really dirty animals? Not at all; just think of them as misunderstood.

When they aren't scarfing down whatever they can find in the wild, pigs on most modern-day farms are fed an energy-rich diet of grains, proteins, vitamins, minerals, and water in order to make them suitable for market. Hogs marketed in the United States consume six to eight pounds of feed per day by the time they reach market weight. Today, most farm-raised hogs are kept in controlled environments and given feed that is made primarily from corn and soybean products, along with a mineral pack that promotes strong bones capable of supporting the pig's muscle weight. Perhaps this is a more civilized and cost-efficient approach, but it's certainly not as much fun as the mud and slop!

Increasing demand for higher quality pork has led to the growth of a niche pork industry that focuses on raising pigs through a more natural—and some would say humane—approach that results in richer flavors and better fat content. They are, essentially, free-range pigs. These pigs are raised in outdoor pastures using methods that are actually based on the way pigs were raised before large-scale farms became commonplace. The free-rangers' feed does not contain some of the antibiotics and supplements that are sometimes found in the feed of a larger farm. Some people believe that in addition to creating tastier meat, hogs from farms with a free-range approach are not subjected to the stress they may experience in a "confinement operation," the industry term for keeping the pigs in custom-constructed buildings where temperature, humidity, and feeding methods are controlled. Advocates of the free-range approach believe the happier the pig is, the happier we'll be with our bacon.

While still not as commonly available as bacon from hogs raised in a confinement operation, bacon from free-range hogs is becoming more readily available over the Internet and through specialty grocery stores. Niman Ranch, based in Northern California but with producers throughout the Midwest, has been raising pigs using celebrated organic methods since the 1970s. Today their operation has grown to include more than 500 independent family farmers, which makes them the largest producer of niche pork in the United States. That's a lot of happy hogs.

However, the majority of pigs raised for market today come from confinement operations concentrated in a few key regions of the United States. These large-scale operations continue to be the primary source of the bacon that is so readily available at the grocery store. And I think we can all agree that having ready access to bacon is very, very, *very* important.

FARM TO MARKET

We humans have an odd habit of anthropomorphizing animals, including the animals that end up on our plates for dinner. Even the most pork-loving of us feels a slight twinge of guilt eating a slice of bacon after watching Wilbur defy his destiny in *Charlotte's Web*. But the fact remains that your breakfast bacon does come from a cute, cuddly piglet that was once wallowing in mud or commiserating with fellow swine in a pen. Most pigs are marked for slaughter from birth, and their choice meats will eventually find their way to your local supermarket. So if you're into eating bacon, you have to swallow the fact that it comes from one of Wilbur's cousins.

So what's it like on a farm where spiders aren't leading a "save the pig" campaign? It's a bit more sophisticated these days than the way old MacDonald might have done things on his farm, and many hog farmers have had to adapt to the changing market in recent years. Like many hog farmers today, Steve Wesley of Waterville, Minnesota, has been in the hog farming business since he was born. "I raised pigs in a straw pile when I was growing up. Back then the hog raising was done by many farmers," according to Steve. "We had fifty sows. We turned a boar out with them in the pasture—some of them had pigs when they came in, some of them had pigs out in a hole in the woods, and some of the pigs were born in a straw pile in the winter. Some froze, some made it. And that's the way it was and everyone did it the same way."

Then the hog farming business began to change and when the sows looked like they were about to have babies, Steve would bring them in and put them in pens. That way they got more piglets out of the sow and had more to sell.

But just when the Wesleys thought they had things figured out, the hog farming business changed yet again. The sows were kept in pens until they were impregnated, at which point they were moved to crates so they wouldn't crush the piglets after giving birth. Heat lamps helped to keep the baby pigs warm. "So that process went along really well for us for quite a few years," Steve said. "And then the pig business changed again. And this time it changed seriously." The down-home business of hog farming was about to go big time.

As the hog farming industry started consolidating into a smaller group of larger players, small producers had to adjust to survive. The Wesleys joined with other farmers to create a larger co-op unit. This may have taken some of the charm out of the original approach to raising pigs in a picturesque open pasture, but the improvements have helped these family-run businesses survive. Steve explains that he and his wife now work with a larger group of eighty producers in a co-op that collectively has 16,000 sows. Every eight weeks pigs from the co-op are dropped off and the Wesleys feed them, take care of them, sell them, and then restock. "And that's the way society wants it to be now. We were on our own, but the packer wants every pig to be exactly the same. If they're going to have it exactly the same, then every pig needs to come from the gene pool, has to be fed the same, raised the same." So these days Wilbur may look just like Tom, Dick, or Harry, but he's still "some pig" (and one that will eventually make "some bacon lovers" very happy).

Most hog farmers now use a genetics company that produces that genetically modified Super Pig. The gene pool is researched by the company and they produce the stock that is sent to the farm to breed the sows. The goal is to breed with the genetically best possible boar for that sow. Creepy? Maybe. Unromantic? Sure. But the customer gets what the customer demands.

The ultimate goal for today's hog farmer is to raise an animal that can live, eat feed, and not have disease problems. A lot of diseases can now be dealt with genetically, allowing the use of minimal antibiotics. According to Wesley, "We will give an injection to a pig that is sick, but that pig has to go for a certain amount of time without antibiotics or we won't be able to sell it. And now most of our vaccines are in the water. The pigs just drink it, gain immunity, and away they go!"

The adjustments to the gene pool over time have made things more efficient for today's hog farmers. Whereas before it took five pounds of feed to produce one pound of pork, thanks to genetics now the ratio is two to one. It's easier to put on a pound of lean than a pound of fat. The pigs are raised this way because the average consumer wants bacon to be leaner with less fat. But these changes have resulted in an animal that would no longer survive out in the straw pile, the way pigs were raised fifty years ago. Because the pigs are so lean, they have no fat or cover on them to keep warm. These sows and boars could never live outside; to accommodate their need for a warmer climate (and because a trip to Miami is out of the question), barns are now temperature-controlled. The genetics may make better bacon, but there's no more fun playing in the snow for these pigs.

BAC'N BITS

"I Smell Bacon"

When used as slang, this is a term to describe the nearby presence of cops. When used in a literal sense, this saying is often followed by "and it smells delicious!" The phrase was also popularized in the commercial for Beggin' Strips dog treats.

"Save One's Bacon"

This phrase was originally used to describe escaping a situation without injury, particularly to the backside where someone was most likely to be beaten. Now the saying is used in a broader sense to describe avoiding a precarious situation.

"When Pigs Fly"

This phrase for describing when something is unlikely to occur is said to be a centuries-old Scottish proverb. It was also popularized in *Alice in Wonderland* when Alice was told by the Duchess that she has just as much of a right to think "as pigs have to fly."

"Living High on the Hog"

Pigs are at their happiest when they are rolling around in the mud, gorging on slop, and enjoying a complete and fulfilling life of barnyard activities. We humans are equally happy when we are "living high on the hog" and experiencing all that life has to offer.

"Go Hog Wild"

The exact origin of "going hog wild" is unknown, but if you've ever eaten more than a pound of bacon in one sitting, then you are probably familiar with the concept.

Some states are now passing laws to do away with crating of sows. Most of these efforts are being led by animal rights activists. But again, because of genetic improvements, most pigs on large-scale farms today wouldn't survive outside. So if the laws change, then hog farmers like the Wesleys will have to change the genetics of their swine. They'd have to revert to the old breeds. All of this is possible, but consumers shouldn't underestimate the impact this would have on the price of their bacon when contemplating such issues in the voting booth.

DOING THE DEED

Raising a hog for market begins long before birth. Sows are typically impregnated through artificial insemination, which is not a terribly romantic undertaking, but it is much more efficient for the farmer than waiting until the "moment is right."

Even with artificial insemination, boars still play a role on the farm. They are trained to walk up and down in front of the sows to show who is in heat. Their whole day is spent walking around the barn talking to the girls. Sounds like a pretty good life, right, boys? The boars are let loose in the morning, escorted by a note-taker. As the boar strolls by, the sows might show signs such as vocalization, "flirting" with their ears, responding to pressure on their rump, and swollen pig-lady bits. Sounds like your average night at the local pub, right? If a sow has any of these reactions, her number is written down. After dinner the number is transferred to the people who come in and do the inseminating ("Hey, baby, call me!"). The next morning, the whole courting process starts all over again.

Once the deed is done, the gestation period is 114 days. The sows are closely monitored during that period of time to minimize stress and complications. No pesky boys or cranky roommates allowed! The sow then typically delivers—or "farrows"—an average of ten young per litter. The farrowing takes place in a pen or stall that protects both newborn pigs and workers. The primary goal is to protect the piglets from accidentally being crushed by the sow. The baby pigs are monitored to minimize mortality and ensure proper early growth.

The piglets are weaned after about three weeks. At this point they weigh between ten and fifteen pounds. They say bye-bye to mama and off they go. The piglets are moved to a nursery—also called a wean-finish building—where they are fed a special diet to assist their development. The piglets get to hang out and play in the nursery for a few weeks. They live the footloose and fancy-free lifestyle of a piglet until they reach a hefty fifty pounds, at which point they're moved into the adult population. Then playtime is over, and it's time to get down to the serious business of packing on the pounds.

Once the pig has been moved to a "finishing farm," they grow to a market weight of between 250 and 270 pounds. On an organic farm, the finishing process might involve feeding the pigs a special diet of acorns or other natural foods to further develop the pig's fat content. Either way, the finishing process is where that luscious balance of fat and lean is developed to make our precious bacon. According to Herb Eckhouse, whose company La Quercia makes high-quality Italian-style cured meats in Des Moines, Iowa, acorn-fed pigs create a meat that is really creamy. "It has an unbelievably silky texture. It carries flavor really well." Ronny Drennan of Broadbent Hams in Kuttawa, Kentucky, agrees, "It's a lot fatter. It does have a really good flavor. I won't say it's a better flavor, it's just fatter. And fat tends to carry the flavor more than the lean." Regardless of how the hog is finished, the process takes place either in an enclosed controlled environment, a partially open facility, or a pasture, depending on the approach the particular farmer takes. The end result is a beautiful, full-bellied hog that so graciously provides us with the delicious pork products we desire.

The entire farrow-to-finish process takes about twenty-six weeks on average (sometimes longer for organically raised swine). Can you imagine going from zero to 250 pounds in just twenty-six weeks? Talk about living high on the hog. The finished hogs are then sold either at a live-weight market or auction, or on a live-weight or carcass-weight basis directly to packers. More than 70 percent of pigs in the United States are now sold on a carcass-pricing system by which the price is determined by particular characteristics of the animal. Once the sales transaction is complete, the hogs then move on to their "final destination."

Describing the slaughter process is kind of tricky, since there is no delicate way of explaining it. But carnivorous humans must accept that in order for us to have access to the delectable pork products we so highly covet, an animal's life must be taken. It is part of the natural order. So if you have a weak stomach, you may want to skip ahead to the next section.

It's important to note that while small organic farms treat their pigs differently than confinement operations during the process of raising pigs for market, the fundamentals of the slaughter process are pretty much the same regardless of the size of your operation (thanks largely to the efforts of your friendly neighborhood USDA inspector). Here's what happens: At the processing facility, the pigs enter a pen called a lairage, and are inspected for any disease or irregularities. While pigs are in lairage, the goal is to make the transition to the afterlife as pain-free as possible for them. It is also beneficial from a business perspective to keep the situation stress-free, because stress can negatively affect the quality of the meat. Stress affects the glycogen levels in the animal's body, which in turn affects the pH levels in the muscle. If the pH levels are off, the pork producer will wind up with either dark, dry meat or pale, watery meat. Neither one is good eating.

After a couple of hours in stress-free lairage, the pigs are moved to a stunning pen where they are rendered unconscious by an electric current sent directly to the brain. The good news is that stunning is reported to be pain-free and, even better, the pigs never see it coming. The pigs are then hung and slaughtered by penetrating the neck artery. The blood is drained and typically preserved for later use in food production. Vampires aren't the only ones with a taste for blood: blood sausage, also known as black pudding, is a celebrated culinary icon in many cultures. The hide is then de-haired, which is done by first scalding the carcass with hot water, then putting it through a de-hairing machine, and finally singeing the remaining hairs.

After being scraped and brushed, the carcass is then opened at the front and the innards—tongue, heart, lungs, liver, stomach, etc.—are removed. The pig is again inspected, weighed, measured, and moved to a chilling room. During the chilling process, the carcass is cooled to between 40 and 45 degrees Fahrenheit within twenty-four hours of being slaughtered. The lower temperature prevents bacterial growth, and also aids the process of cutting the meat.

One day after being slaughtered, the carcass is ready to be butchered. First the head and feet are removed. The pig is divided into five parts: shoulder butt, picnic shoulder, loin, leg (ham), and side/belly. The meat is then ready to be distributed. The pork belly is on its way to becoming a dreamy slab of bacon.

(If you chose not to risk the possibility of your passion for pork products being diminished by learning about the details of pig slaughter, you can safely resume reading here.)

WHY IS BACON SO DELICIOUS?

There are dozens of ways a pig can be consumed, and every single one is worthwhile. The most common cuts are belly (where The Best Meat Ever comes from), ham, ribs, shoulder butt, sausage, loin, roast, and chops. Even trotters (aka pigs' feet), ears, and tails can be eaten. There are also many uses for pork by-products, including replacement heart valves, pharmaceuticals, skin grafts, insulin, cement, insulation, upholstery, antifreeze, rubber, explosives, soap, chalk, brushes, fertilizer, insecticides, fabric dye, gelatin, glue, plastics, cosmetics . . . you name it, a pig has probably contributed to it. And that list just scratches the surface. Needless to say, from a cost-benefit perspective, pigs are a tremendously valuable animal.

Humans have been curing pork for consumption for thousands of years, but use of the term "bacon" to describe cured pork belly wasn't applied until much later. The word "bacon" originated from words in Old German (*bakkon*) and Old French (*bako*). "Bacon" or "bacoun" first appeared in the English language around the twelfth century, initially to describe pork in general. A few hundred years later, "bacon" began to describe the cured pork belly we know and love today.

Bacon is cut from the pig's side, belly, and back. To understand why bacon is so delicious, it's important to understand these parts of the pig. The thick strips of fat and lean streaks of meat in these areas are what give bacon its familiar marbled appearance and—most important—why it has such a distinctly appealing taste when cured. The layers allow the meat and fat to absorb the right amount of salt and smoke to give bacon its perfect flavor balance. This is the central reason why bacon is so incredibly tasty.

There are several ways to cure meat, but the oldest and most common method for making bacon is salt curing. Not only does a salt cure create the addictively familiar flavor of bacon but it also helps to prevent bacterial growth and slows down the process of spoilage. Salt is such a powerful preserving agent that it's no wonder it was used as currency in ancient times. Bacon preserved up until the early 1900s contained far more salt than the version we purchase from the supermarket today. Modern-day packaging and refrigeration help to preserve meat longer at a lower sodium level, which is important in terms of diminishing its impact on blood pressure and dehydration. Most important: less sodium means we get to eat more bacon!

Smoking is another method of preserving bacon. Smoking helps to prevent bacterial growth, but more important, it adds color and flavor. While not all salt-cured bacon is smoked, almost all smoked bacon first goes through a salt cure for purposes of preservation. Hickory-smoked and applewood-smoked bacon are two varieties commonly available in grocery stores.

There's a movement afoot among food enthusiasts to cure and smoke their own bacon at home, which can be fun. These impressively ambitious people like the adventure of making their own bacon and putting their own personal twist on traditional methods handed down through generations. Other people prefer to leave this task to the professionals. Either way, the endgame for all of us is to gain access to as much bacon as possible.

THE BACON REVOLUTION

Like Americans, the British have long consumed bacon and eggs for breakfast. This is not surprising, as so much of our culinary tradition stems from our origins as an outpost of the British empire. The Brits, bless their hearts, were among the first to refine the process of curing bacon for commercial purposes. John Harris, a butcher in Wiltshire, England, in the 1770s, led this charge. The pig trade that existed at the time between Ireland and England made Wiltshire a stopover for pigs being herded from the port town of Bristol to London, where they were sold at Smithfield, an area of northwest London that has served as a meat market for more than 800 years. Harris ran a feeding and resting station and was able to purchase quality pigs, which frequently wound up as bacon in the process. But the Harris family fun didn't stop there. When the pig trade declined significantly during the potato famine in the mid-1800s, Harris's great-grandson took a trip to America to look into the possibility of importing pigs. Instead he came back with the brilliant idea of building an icehouse in which he could keep butchered pigs fresh for longer periods of time. With an icehouse, the Harris family could cure bacon year round. Thus the Harris Bacon Company was founded. Harris Bacon operated in Wiltshire well into the twentieth century.

The British affinity for bacon by no means begins or ends with the Harris clan. Not to be outdone by other cultures that might celebrate marital bliss with flowers and elaborate cakes, the Brits manage to throw a little bacon into the mix. Starting back in the twelfth century, the tradition of the Dunmow Flitch Trial came into existence. The trial is essentially a ceremony, started in the town of Dunmow, in which a prize is given to any married man who could swear before a congregation and God that he had not quarreled with his wife for a year and a day. The prize was a "flitch," a side of bacon. As a testament to the enduring appeal of bacon, the flitch trials still take place today, with couples staying on their best behavior in hopes of getting their hands on—and teeth into—their salty reward. This is another rumored source of the saying "bringing home the bacon."

It bears mentioning that the English do have slightly different terminology for their beloved bacon. While we refer to slices of bacon, the English call each individual strip a rasher, while a whole side of bacon is a gammon. Although the origin of these words has been somewhat lost to time, theories abound. The more commonly used "rasher" is believed to have come into general usage in England in the mid-sixteenth century, and is derived from the now obsolete term "rase," which means "to shave." Which is how you get your slice, or rasher, to come off the belly or back in those nice thin strips. Whatever you decide to call it, it's always delightful.

Much like the English, the Danes were also quick to catch on to the concept of curing bacon for commercial purposes. In the mid-1800s, grain imported to Denmark from North America was quite cheap and Danish farmers began to diversify their crops with a heavier focus on pork production. In 1847, the first exports of Danish bacon to the United Kingdom were shipped, a practice that grew exponentially over the next several decades. To this day, Danish bacon is still the most popular bacon in England.

BACON FOR THE MASSES

Prior to the introduction of prepackaged bacon in the United States, consumers either raised their own pigs to cure their own bacon, or they bought bacon from butchers, typically by the slab. Prepackaged, presliced bacon was introduced in the United States in 1924 by Oscar Mayer, an immigrant from Bavaria who had opened a meat-packing business in Chicago with his brothers in the late 1800s.

Oscar Mayer's first bacon packaging featured shingled slices, wrapped in cellophane and placed in a cardboard frame—an idea for which the company holds the original U.S. patent. With this clever invention, Oscar Mayer went from being a minor bacon producer to a top brand, a status it still maintains to this day. They also hold the distinction of being the only meat production company in the United States whose name is a favorite childhood jingle for kids to sing as they scarf down bacon, bologna, and hot dogs. Behold, the power of meat and marketing.

Other major bacon brands in the United States today are Smith-field and Hormel. Smithfield Foods is named after the town in which the company is headquartered: Smithfield, Virginia. Smithfield is the largest hog producer and pork processor in the world, with facilities in the United States, Canada, France, Poland, and Japan. Smithfield offers dozens of bacon options under the brand names Smithfield, Lykes, Sunnyland, Jamestown, Gwaltney, Aberdeen, Blueridge, Esskay, Reelfoot, and Valleydale. Something for everyone. If you take a trip to your local supermarket today, chances are very good that you would encounter a Smithfield brand of bacon. If not, you're just not looking hard enough.

Hormel has also been makin' bacon for more than a hundred years. Hormel's Black Label line has long been recognized for its high quality. The Black Label moniker is actually an idea that was borrowed from Johnny Walker scotch, another black-labeled product with a loyal following. At some point along the way, black labels came to be known as representing ultrapremium status. And for this reason, Hormel bacon can be found in the freezers of many bacon fanatics. Like many bacon producers, Hormel also produces a fully cooked bacon product. The bacon has been cooked and just needs to be warmed in the microwave (or it can even be eaten cold). It's not exactly the most appetizing form of bacon money can buy—but convenience does rule the day for a lot of people and this particular product is quickly gaining in popularity.

In addition to the major producers, there are countless independent producers who sell their artisanal bacons through specialty stores, at farmers' markets, and over the Internet. Most small producers are relatively unknown to the general public, yet they create some of the best bacon available today. Some producers even have a cult-like following of chefs and consumers who crave bacon the way it is meant to be cured—with a lot of love and attention to detail that can't be easily replicated in a factory.

Bacon is making more frequent appearances on the menus of some of the top restaurants in the country, and much of the bacon those restaurants serve comes from the smaller, independent producers who sell better cuts of meat richer in flavor than the bacon that can be bought in the supermarket. Those quality cuts and cures are inspiring chefs to serve bacon in some incredibly unique and inventive ways.

CHAPTER 2

THE ART OF MAKIN' BACON

"Pig—let me speak his praise—is no less provocative of the
appetite, than he is satisfactory to the criticalness of the
censorious palate. The strong man may batten on him, and
the weakling refuseth not his mild juices."
—*A Dissertation Upon Roast Pig*
by Charles Lamb

E VERYTHING ABOUT SWINE is divine. There really isn't a part of
the pig that isn't delicious. But let's get real . . . bacon is, without
question, the most popular food product to come from the humble
pig. It could easily be argued that among the pork-loving population,
a significant majority always has at least one package of bacon in their
freezer at home. The same can't be said for ribs, ham, and chops, no
matter how much we love them. A slow-roasted suckling pig is one
of the best culinary delights in the world, but you can't just keep one
hanging around the house until the time is right for a hog roast. Bacon, on the other hand, is an everyday meat that can be stored in your
refrigerator or freezer for long periods of time with minimal impact
on the quality of the meat. Bacon is the King of Pork. Bacon is The
Best Meat Ever.

BACON MAKES THE WORLD GO ROUND

There are hundreds of bacon varieties to choose from. And the kind
of bacon you're familiar with even depends on where you live in the
world. In the United States alone, there are multiple options. The bacon most Americans dream of eating for breakfast on Sunday morning typically comes from the belly of the pig. But Americans might
also encounter a strain called Kansas City bacon at their local butcher,
which comes from the shoulder. Some country-style smokehouses
produce a product called country ham bacon which is actually lean
ham sliced thin like bacon. In the United Kingdom, Ireland, Austra-
lia, and New Zealand, American-style bacon is referred to as "streaky"
bacon, and is less common than the back bacon rasher they are more
familiar with, which comes from the loin. In the United States, we
know back bacon as Canadian bacon, which Canadians call peameal

bacon. Pork jowl can also be cured as a bacon-like product (known as *guanciale* in Italy). And speaking of Italy, we can't forget *pancetta*, bacon's half-sibling. As you can see, there are many different kinds of bacon, and it can be really confusing to keep track of all the options available to you!

In the same way that the word "bacon" doesn't mean the same thing everywhere in the English-speaking world, the word "speck" also creates cross-cultural confusion. *Speck* is the direct German translation of the word "bacon." But throughout German-speaking Europe and Italy, *speck* often refers to a type of prosciutto. *Speck dell'Alto Adige* (*Südtiroler Speck*) is one of the most celebrated forms of prosciutto. And in Germany, speck is also sometimes a product that is more like Italian lardo, which is cured fatback. *Sprechen sie bacon?!?* English speakers aren't the only ones creating confusion when it comes to cured pork products.

Access to a variety of bacon products isn't just limited to westerners. Asian cultures are equally enamored with all things swine. The Chinese have been enjoying cured pork for thousands of years, and they indulge in a bacon-like product called *lop yuk*. Lop yuk is made by curing pork belly with soy sauce, brown sugar, and spices. Sometimes it is also smoked. Their next door neighbors in Korea take pleasure in a bacon treat called *samgyeopsal*. Also made from cured pork belly, the word "samgyeopsal" translates into "three-layered meat"—an obvious reference to the profile of a sliced pork belly. This author once had the opportunity to sample this delicacy at a restaurant in Beijing owned by the North Korean government. Despite being an incredibly bizarre dining adventure, the samgyeopsal was delicious and a culinary high point of the "dining for Dear Leader" experience.

A SALTY SOLUTION

Regardless of where you live and what your bacon looks like, the curing process is the underlying concept that unites bacon around the world. Not all bacon is smoked, but almost all bacon is cured one way or another. And the curing process makes the meat more receptive to the smoking process. Can you imagine if our ancestors had never figured out that salt is the perfect curing agent? Can you imagine a world without bacon? It's sad to even contemplate. We should make a toast to salt and our super-great-grandparents every time we lift a juicy strip of bacon to our lips.

Salt curing is one of the oldest forms of food preservation. Before the nineteenth century, refrigeration wasn't a reliable or affordable way for most people to prevent food spoilage. In our quest to maintain our status at the top of the food chain, humans eventually figured out that salt prevents bacterial growth and allows perishable food to be stored for longer periods of time while minimizing waste. That a salt cure can also make meat more tasty was just an added bonus.

These days most of us take for granted the process a pork belly must go through in order to be cured and delivered to our local grocery store. But there are many ways to cure bacon, and it's worth understanding the different approaches because they all produce a different version of The Best Meat Ever. Bacon can be either dry cured or wet cured. The dry cure method is the oldest form of curing—it is the life-changing approach our ancestors developed thousands of years ago (for which we thank them every morning). A typical basic dry cure is made with salt and sugar (the sugar counteracts the harshness of the salt). The cure mixture also sometimes contains sodium nitrite (aka pink salt) and/or sodium nitrate (aka saltpeter), and if desired, seasonings to give the bacon a characteristic flavor. Sounds complicated, right? It's actually not that difficult. But just to make things a bit more confusing, a dry cure is also sometimes referred to as a sugar cure, which doesn't seem to make much sense given that the primary ingredient of the curing mixture is salt. But the sugar reference is meant to distinguish the dry cure from a straight salt cure, which is how most bacon was cured prior to the twentieth century. Most citizens of the twenty-first century would gag if they were to eat a strip of the salt-cured bacon of a hundred years ago. Fortunately, bacon has evolved along with civilization and our bacon no longer tastes like a salt lick.

Wet cures (also called a wet brine or sweet pickle brine) are more common with today's mass-market bacon producers. This form of curing was developed in the United Kingdom in the nineteenth century by the Harris family, one of the first producers of bacon for the masses and true visionaries of the early Bacon Nation. A wet cure is conducted by immersing the meat in a liquid brine (a solution made with salt, sodium nitrite, sugar, and water) and refrigerating it for three to four days. Instead of submerging the belly in the liquid brine, industrial producers usually inject the pork belly with the brine solution—aka "Botox for bacon."

While we're on the subject of all the additives that are part of the process of makin' bacon, we might take a moment to discuss substances that have bedeviled the bacon's reputation for quite some time. That's right, we're talking about sodium nitrite and sodium nitrate. What is this stuff, and why does it make some people so nervous?

Sodium nitrite and sodium nitrate are key components in the process of curing meats for commercial purposes. The two ingredients combine with the meat's myoglobin to give it that desirable reddish-pinkish color we all associate with healthy meat. But in addition, sodium nitrite supposedly prevents bacterial growth and retards rancidity (facts debated by some). Sodium nitrite is sometimes referred to as "pink salt" because of the color added to the salt in order to prevent it from being confused with table salt when you are cooking at home. You definitely wouldn't want to sprinkle this stuff on top of the food on your dinner plate. Salt is good, but not when it requires a trip to the emergency room.

Nitrites and nitrates can be found naturally in our environment. Two of Earth's most common elements, nitrogen and oxygen, combine to form these nitrogen-containing compounds. Nitrates and nitrites are essential nutrients for plants to grow, and can be found in the air, soils, surface waters, and underground drinking water. Doesn't sound so bad, right?

However, high doses of nitrites and nitrates can be toxic. A serving of bacon doesn't contain anything close to a lethal dose (which, for you *CSI* fans, is about 22 milligrams per kilogram of body weight). To reach a dangerous level, a person would need to consume more than eighteen pounds of bacon in one sitting. Even if some daring person was able to accomplish that lofty goal, they are more likely to die from other factors—including a salt overdose—than they would from nitrite poisoning.

But because these products are potentially toxic to humans, the federal government regulates the amount that can be used during the commercial curing process. Additionally, even though potassium nitrate (also called saltpeter) has historically been the primary ingredient used for curing meats, now sodium nitrite in combination with sodium nitrate is most commonly used. There are several premixed products available to consumers who cure their own bacon at home to prevent accidental overdose.

Since questions have been raised about the impact of sodium nitrite and sodium nitrate on human beings, some companies that produce bacon have removed these ingredients from their curing process entirely. Beyond the aforementioned potential health concerns, there is a small percentage of the population who are allergic to nitrates and for whom nitrate-free bacon is the only way to enjoy The Best Meat Ever. Uncured bacon is becoming more commonly available in grocery stores. Other producers are exploring the preservation of bacon through "natural" methods such as celery juice (which, incongruously, also contains a certain level of nitrates). However, the majority of large commercial bacon producers still use these products—but as mentioned, they are heavily regulated by the government, so you don't need to worry about whether or not your bacon is going to kill you when you're deciding which type to purchase at the grocery store. Enough said.

HOT SMOKING VERSUS COLD SMOKING

While both the curing and smoking processes give bacon a distinctive flavor, it's the smoking that really gets most bacon fanatics excited about their favorite breakfast meat. Smoking is what gives the meat that earthy scent and flavor that engenders the primal human attraction to food cooked over a fire. Smoking also plays a role in preventing spoilage. During the smoking process, chemicals are added to the surface of the bacon, making it more difficult for bacteria to develop and penetrate the meat. But the best feature of the smoke is that it creates a lovely scent that penetrates every corner of your home when you're frying bacon on a Sunday morning and it has the power to coax even the most morning-hating person out of bed.

So what exactly does it mean for bacon to be smoked? Technically speaking, smoking is the process of cooking meat by exposing it to smoke from a burning substance in some sort of enclosed structure. For the individual making his or her own bacon at home, this structure may be a homemade smoking device fashioned from a non-galvanized garbage can (a little bit "trashy" but effective), a barbecue grill (for the fierce suburban warrior), or a professional electric smoker (for the home cook who just doesn't screw around with their meat-smoking projects). For bacon producers, smoking usually takes place in a smokehouse, which is an entire room or building dedicated to this process. Now that you know what goes on in the smokehouse, let's all agree that it should be treated with the same level of reverence as any house of worship. If not, you may want to reconsider the depth of your love for bacon. Just saying.

There are two ways to smoke meat: cold smoking and hot smoking. Hot smoking is actually cooking meat over a fire, typically for purposes of consuming the meat immediately after it is done. If you've barbecued a delicious bacon-wrapped steak on an outdoor grill, then you're a hot smokin' pro. But how in the world can something be cold-smoked over a hot fire? Cold smoking might not be as familiar to the average person, but this is the all-important process used to smoke bacon. Cold smoking is done over several hours or days, and the food being smoked is only subjected to the smoke from the fire, not the actual fire. As a result, the food isn't actually cooked—nothing about the texture of the food changes through cold smoking. Only the flavors change. And they change in a really, really good way.

Many different kinds of wood can be used to smoke bacon. The ones most commonly used are hickory, apple, alder, cherry, oak, maple, mesquite, pecan, and beech. When burnt, each of these woods gives bacon a distinctive flavor that also varies depending on the length of time the meat is smoked. It's this sweet, smoky flavor combined with the saltiness of the cured bacon that appeals to the most basic of human desires.

If the salt cure and smoking process don't do enough for bacon to arouse your senses, there are also many specialty flavors to choose from. Bacon producers are regularly using flavors such as pepper, cinnamon, paprika, garlic, and jalapeño to enhance their bacon. Father's Country Hams in Bremen, Kentucky, is not only one of the oldest and best producers of country-style bacon in the United States but they also have the widest and most varied selection of flavored bacons available to consumers today. Some of their flavors include apple-cinnamon, blueberry-cinnamon, Cajun, jalapeño, peach-cinnamon, vanilla-bourbon, and honey BBQ, among others. Father's is truly leading the way when it comes to all of the ways you can flavor bacon for a different twist on The Best Meat Ever. Another unusual flavor on the market is a sun-dried tomato–flavored bacon from Broadbent Hams in Kuttawa, Kentucky. If you opt to make your own bacon at home, you could use pretty much any favorite spice or flavor to enhance your bacon eating experience. The possibilities are endless and are completely dependent on your own secret porky fantasies.

INVESTING IN THE FUTURE WITH BACON

Pork belly futures have been traded at the Chicago Mercantile Exchange since 1961 and are based on the current supply of frozen pork bellies compared to anticipated demand. As our demand for delicious bacon increases, so does the value of pork bellies. With bacon being as popular as it is right now, and showing no signs of waning, investing in pork belly futures is a sound financial decision.

MOMMY, WHERE DOES BACON COME FROM?

Have you ever paused to wonder what journey your bacon went through to reach your breakfast plate? Perhaps the pleasing aroma and seductive taste of bacon is too overwhelming for you to think about anything other than inhaling it as quickly as possible, so maybe you haven't thought much about it. And thanks to the easy access we have to a wide selection of bacon options at the grocery store, most of us don't have to think much about how it got to us in the first place. But there's an entire industry behind each package of lovingly cured and smoked bacon, and it's an industry full of people who are obsessed with bacon just as much as you are.

The bacon most consumers eat today is made by large corporate producers such as Smithfield, Hormel, and Oscar Mayer, and is sold at pretty much every supermarket in the United States. But like many independent bacon producers today, even these large players started out by paying their dues and earning respect for their products as smaller independent producers. For example, Hormel has been making bacon since 1891. According to Jason Baskin, an associate product manager at Hormel Foods, their company started out small. The founder, George Hormel, used to personally trim every single bacon slab himself to ensure uniform excellence. Today Hormel is one of the largest bacon producers in the world, and their process is highly automated, but the basic concepts for making good bacon are the same as they were when Hormel was just a neighborhood operation. Find some good pork bellies, cure and smoke them with love, and the result will always be a happy human belly.

Despite the market dominance of the large bacon producing companies, numerous independent country-style smokehouses all over the United States are still doing quite well at making and selling artisanal bacon to a smaller but highly fanatical market that craves the traditional flavor of bacon.

Country-style hams and bacon are made all over the United States, but some of the best bacon in the world comes from producers in Tennessee, Kentucky, and Missouri. A lot of people say this area of the United States is ideal for curing meat because of the year-round temperatures and humidity there. Most smokehouses today have artificial temperature control, but there was a time when they didn't have that option. Before artificial temperature control, the weather was too cold in the northern United States, too warm in the South, and too warm *and* dry out west. Bacon won't take the salt if it's too cold. And if it's too warm it will spoil. Bacon may be delicious, but it sure is finicky! So the tradition of making country-style hams and bacon has been alive and well in Kentucky, Missouri, and Tennessee for generations. Most bacon producers in this part of the country also think there is just something special in the air—that the magical environment is conducive to producing the best possible bacon.

The best thing about a trip through bacon country is that you get to sample lots and lots of bacon, and at the end of the day your clothes and car smell like a smokehouse. Animals will be automatically drawn to your scent. But despite the side effects, a tour of smokehouses in this corner of the United States will give you a real sense of the different approaches to makin' bacon, from the smallest family-owned smokehouses to larger operations with a national customer base. No matter the size of the operation, these businesses all aspire to make the highest quality country-smoked bacon your hard-earned paycheck can buy (just don't spend it all in one place—there are lots of different kinds of bacon to try). Following are profiles of select producers who are making some of the most popular country-style bacon in the United States, whether it's in a brick building in their backyard or a state-of-the-art facility. Each one is unique, but they're all obsessed with producing The Best Meat Ever.

Bacon Just Like Granddad Used to Make

Since 1965, Leslie and June Scott have been making country hams on a property where their home also sits, in a beautiful rural area of western Kentucky with rolling green hills and peaceful pastoral views. The Scotts always had hogs that they slaughtered to make hams and bacon for their family, but gradually a few people from town asked if they could buy hams from them. So eventually they cleaned up an outbuilding to use for producing their hams, and operated their business from the space for about ten years. Thus proving that if you build it, they will come.

The Scotts' ham business became increasingly popular and after a while some of their customers started asking for bacon. "We had built a building by then because the USDA won't let you do it in a chicken coop, so to speak!" says June. (So picky, those USDA inspectors.) The Scotts looked at their building and thought it wouldn't take much room to put twenty-five sides of bacon in there. "And we could make a little money off each one and it might be enough to pay the light bill!"

Initially the Scotts had only intended to sell their sides of bacon whole. According to June, "At first no one asked us to slice it, because that's what they were used to." But because of the changing market with more mothers going into the workforce, it wasn't long before people wanted the Scotts to slice their bacon for them. So they invested in a slicer and vacuum machine and the business took off.

The Scotts never intended for their business to grow to the point that it has today, but given the quality of their product, their success isn't surprising. Because they've done so well, Scott Hams could have looked at other ways to expand their business, but instead they decided to stay small and focused. Their production facility and smokehouse is still a relatively small brick building next door to their house.

Given the remote country location of Scott Hams, most of their products are shipped—as is the case with many smokehouses in this part of the country. To say this area of the United States is "off the beaten path" would be an understatement. "Probably about one third of what we do goes out in gift boxes at Christmas. We advertise a little in the local papers and get some business that way. We also participate in bacon-of-the-month clubs."

Scott Hams is one of the country smokehouses that chooses not to use those big bad scary nitrates. "We've never used nitrates. Our parents didn't. We didn't even really know what it was." Their bacon has a brown cast, while if it had nitrates in it, it would be bright red. "But it doesn't affect the shelf life. I generally tell my customers to keep it for three to four months in the refrigerator, and for a year or so in the freezer. Someone once told me that he had some of our bacon laying on a filing cabinet for more than a year at room temperature, and he said it was still fine when he ate it!" That was one adventurous dude, and his experience might have been the exception. Not all bacon can be kept that long—it really does depend on the kind of bacon you're talking about and how it was cured. But Scott Hams cures their bacon the same way people have traditionally cured bacon for thousands of years, and the original reason for curing bacon was to be able to keep it for long periods of time without the meat spoiling. So if bacon is cured the way it's supposed to be, it is a very hardy meat. "I've never had anyone come by and tell me they kept it long enough that it was rancid." And anyone who keeps bacon that long before eating it should be too ashamed to admit it!

To cure their bacon, the Scotts use a very basic mixture of salt and brown sugar. Sugar helps keep the bacon from tasting too salty. They rub the pork bellies with the cure, put them in a bin, and leave them for about a week. Then they wash the bacon, put it on hooks, and hang it on a rack in a cooler to dry. It sits in the cooler at 40 degrees Fahrenheit for a few days. Once the bellies have finished "hanging out," they are ready for the blessed smoke treatment.

The Scotts use hickory wood to smoke their bacon, just like their forefathers. "My dad has a lot of hickory, so we go over and cut the green hickory." The bellies are smoked for about three days until they turn the right color. Next they're left to sit for a few days so the bellies will harden up, and then the Scotts are ready to slice it. From the time a belly comes in the door to when it is sliced and ready to be sold is typically about three weeks. And then it's only a matter of time before that bacon is in the stomachs of the Scotts' devoted followers.

Like many bacon producers in this part of the country, the Scotts get their meat from a company called Premium Standard Farms in Missouri (which is now owned by Smithfield). They buy just the cuts they need to produce their products—bellies and hams. "We buy select. We buy the best they've got. We like our bacon to be nice and lean." Most small bacon producers buy their meat from companies like Premium Standard because it is more efficient than raising their own hogs, which would require building a slaughter facility and finding a use for all parts of the pig—something that would be quite difficult for most small producers to do while staying profitable.

So what is it about country-style bacon that appeals to a certain kind of customer? June Scott thinks it's familiarity. "Many times we hear it's like granddad made on the farm. It must taste a lot like what people made in Appalachia, because we get people from there telling us it's like what they had as a child.

"There's one lady who buys it all the time—she's ninety-something, and she calls Leslie 'the boy' and every time she sends her check in she says, 'the boy has done a great job again, it tastes just like grand-daddy's!'" Scott Hams also has a somewhat unusual market in Civil War reenactors who like to buy bacon by the slab. If anything can unite the North and South, it's definitely a delicious slab o' bacon.

Many bacon producers in this part of the country agree that there has been an increased interest in their bacon products in the last five years. The Scotts have experienced this same phenomenon. "It's kind of puzzling. I guess it's because it's something we had as a child. It's just good. It's like all of those people have just now discovered how great bacon is." Whatever the reason, country-style bacon is definitely back in style again.

Above all else, the Scotts just really enjoy making country-style bacon and hams and dealing with customers. "People who buy country ham and bacon are nice and honest," says June. And understandably that's enough to get the Scotts out of bed and into the smokehouse each morning.

The Ham Lady

Like the Scotts, Nancy "The Ham Lady" Newsom Mahaffey, an iconic fixture in Princeton, Kentucky, is producing world-class bacon and ham as a family operation in a humble smokehouse in a small town. And it's clear she's having fun with her booming business. Some of the top restaurants in the country just can't get enough of Nancy's superior cured meats. She's not just The Ham Lady—she's arguably The Ham Queen.

The spelling of Newsom was actually Newsham when the family first moved to the United States in the 1600s. Talk about destiny. They settled in Virginia initially, but eventually made their way to Kentucky for a land grant of 1,600 acres. They brought their ham and bacon curing processes with them. Nancy's grandfather opened a general store in Princeton in 1917 and began selling hams to local customers. Eventually Nancy's father, Colonel Bill Newsom, took over the business and expanded the ham operation. Then in 1975, James Beard wrote an article about him and the business quickly went national.

In 1987, Colonel Newsom was starting to get too old to run the business, and in that same year the building where the store was located in Princeton burned down. At that point Nancy took over the business. Her destiny as The Ham Lady was set; there was no turning back.

Newsom's is best known for their hams, but as with other country ham producers in the area, they've been making and selling bacon for many years as well. According to Nancy, "The key to bacon is to leave it in long enough to cure, but not so long that it's too salty." However, one time when she left the bacon for too long, she ended up turning it into a product called Salty Hog that she sold to customers who prefer the saltier bacon that they knew from growing up in the early 1900s. Only a salty lady like Nancy could turn a salty hog into a salty success.

The Newsom's brick smokehouse is located behind Nancy's parents' house on their property in Princeton. Nancy uses an iron kettle to smoke her bacon and hams with burning wood and damp sawdust to make smoke. "I don't think many people do it in a kettle like this anymore. I just want to do it the way it was intended to be done. I could probably double what I cure and sell it all. But after that, it would get to a point where something would be lost. It would lose its soul."

Movin' On Up from the Backyard to the Big Time

Ronny and Beth Drennan are the proprietors of Broadbent Hams, a relatively small family-run business in Kuttawa, Kentucky. They upgraded to a new, modern facility in 2008 to grow their business and take their bacon makin' potential to the next level while continuing to produce the familiar, country-style product that initially made them so popular.

In visiting multiple smokehouses, it quickly becomes clear that the process is pretty simple and doesn't vary much, regardless of how modern the facility may be. Not only is bacon so incredibly addictive but it's also incredibly easy to make. Like the Scotts, the Drennans hand-rub their pork bellies with salt and sugar, let them cure for a week, and then wash them off and hang them on racks. The temperature in the room is kept at 38 to 40 degrees Fahrenheit so the bellies are easier to slice. Just like humans, when bacon has had a chance to "chill out," it's much easier to work with!

Broadbent Hams uses nitrates in most of their bacon, although they do sell some that is nitrate-free. "When we bought the business, that is what they were doing. It's supposed to kill botulism," says Ronny. "Some people say that botulism isn't a problem, some people say it is, but no one really knows. A lot of people want the nitrates."

One key feature of the new Broadbent facility is their modern smoking machine where they use apple, maple, or hickory wood to smoke their bacon. "We use chips that we put in the machine, hit the switch, and it heats up and creates the smoke. It's probably the most expensive thing in the building!" Their new smoker puts more smoke into the room, making the overall process much quicker than before. Faster smoke equals faster bacon, which is a very good thing.

One of Broadbent's most popular bacon flavors is peppered bacon. Have you ever wondered how those little grains of pepper manage to stay affixed to the bacon without falling off? Maybe it's because the pepper is naturally attracted to the bacon just like humans are. But if you really want to know the science behind it, the process of making pepper bacon is actually pretty simple. Ronny Drennan uses a coarsely ground black pepper. "When we bring the bellies out and wash them after they've cured, when most of the water is dried off but it's tacky, we put the pepper on before we smoke it." It's a simple process with a magnificent result.

Like most businesses in the area, most of Broadbent's business is mail order. That is why the Drennans are constantly looking for ways to improve and differentiate their products in order to keep the bacon-eating masses hungry for more. They do sell to some restaurants, but "most restaurants, unless it's really higher end, are looking for price. A lot of them buy from Sysco or somewhere else and they want paper thin slices. We have a thicker slice."

The Drennans have also noticed an increase in their bacon sales over the last few years. Ronny thinks the media is partially responsible. He also gives credit to fast-food restaurants that are featuring bacon on more menu items. For these reasons, people are starting to think about bacon more and are trying different types. The Bacon Nation is dreaming more about bacon, thinking more about bacon, and eating more bacon, and folks like the Drennans are just doing what they can to keep up with the pace.

If the Bacon is Good, Everything Must Be Good

A few hundred miles down the road in Hermann, Missouri, is the Swiss Meat and Sausage Company. Located about two hours west of

St. Louis, Swiss Meats truly produces some of the best bacon in the world. If you are lucky enough to drop by their store, make sure you have ample cooler space in your car. What starts out as a trip to pick up one or two packets of bacon can quickly turn into two coolers full of several kinds of bacon, containers of potato and bacon salad, several packages of German-style sausages, including varieties made with left-over bacon ends, and perhaps even a treat for Fido.

Mike Sloan is the second generation owner-operator of Swiss Meats, which his father started in 1969. He is very passionate about his business, which he considers a labor of love. Initially the business was focused on custom butchery and processing for local farmers. Like so many communities in this part of the United States, everyone used to have their own hogs and cows, so the Sloans had no reason to sell their own ham or bacon. But in the 1970s, those farmers starting scaling back and dying, and if they sold their farm, most of the time they sold it to a recreational farmer who wasn't going to raise hogs. At that point, Swiss Meats started adding more products to their line, and one of the things they focused on was bacon. "I knew that if we had good bacon, it would draw people for other products because they would get the idea that if our bacon was good, then everything must be good." You can always trust a man who makes good bacon.

Swiss Meats started out with just one type of bacon but later expanded their collection to include honey bacon, apple-cinnamon bacon, pepper bacon, jowl bacon, and a unique product called cottage bacon. In some parts of the country cottage bacon is called hillbilly bacon because it's actually made from pork butt (and because it's also good to eat when you're hiding out at your shack in the hills pickin' at your banjo by the campfire). To make cottage bacon, Mike takes the pork butt, debones it, sugar cures it, hickory smokes it, and then slices it thin for use in sandwiches. The selling point? It tastes like bacon, looks like bacon, but is a little leaner than most bacons, and comes in bigger slices. Take care not to overcook it, though: according to Mike, since it's lean it gets crispy quickly when fried, and if it gets too crispy, it will get tough.

Swiss Meats also makes one of the best forms of nonpork bacon: beef bacon. It's made from a brisket that's sugar cured, hickory smoked, and sliced thin. Beef bacon, like cottage bacon, shouldn't be overcooked (it dries out easily). Beef bacon may never reach the popularity level of pork bacon, but a world where these two forms of cured meat live side by side in harmony is the ideal kind of world to live in.

As the major bacon producers have grown larger, Swiss Meats has had to figure out how to specialize in a niche market. "There are a few meat companies that now control the world market and they control about 95 percent. You have to do something better than what the larger companies do, but on a smaller scale. If you try and compete on a larger scale, you'll fail." Larger companies may control the market, but Swiss Meats controls the hearts of a growing segment of the Bacon Nation.

One of the ways Swiss Meats has differentiated itself is with the addition of state-of-the-art technology. In the old days, they hand-rubbed the cures onto the bacon, which led to inconsistent saltiness. But now they have an automated meat tumbler. "This is a really neat machine. It holds about 600 pounds of bacon. We put the bacon in there, weigh our water, salt, and sugar, and add it to the tumbler." And like an Olympic gymnastics champion, Swiss Meats bacon tumbles its way to a gold medal every time. Swiss Meats uses nitrates in their bacon, but they also make a nitrate-free bacon. "Only 2 to 3 percent of consumers are into nitrate-free bacon, but they also eat green beans out of their gardens and what they don't realize is they are getting more nitrates out of green beans than they are out of bacon."

The tumbling machine not only produces a consistent cure but toss a few flavors in there and the party really gets started. "Depending on what kind of bacon we're making . . . if we're adding the honey bacon we'll add honey granules, for applewood bacon we'll add some concentrated apple juice that will go all the way through the bacon. When we take the applewood bacon out, we hand rub it with cinnamon before it goes to the smokehouse for additional flavor. Or if we're making pepper bacon, we'll use our regular recipe and when we take it out, we'll hand rub it with two different sizes of pepper. One pepper is real small and the other is a little bigger, so you get a mixture of both. It looks nice with a lot of variation." And bacon variety is definitely the spice of life.

So what exactly happens in this magical tumbling machine to make great tasting bacon? When Mike closes the lid and turns the machine on, the vacuum gently pulls the muscles of the meat apart. Then the machine starts rotating, and as it rotates the pieces of bacon will fall and drop and strike against one another. Through a fifteen-hour process, the tumbling motion acts as a mechanical tenderization of the meat, and the vacuum sucks all of the ingredients into the center of the bacon. When you open the door of the machine after fifteen hours and take the meat out, it's bone dry. The water, salt, and seasonings are gone. There's nothing left but cured bacon so good you might be tempted to eat it raw right out of the machine. But most employees of Swiss Meats resist that urge, and instead they take the bacon out, hang it on a rack to let it dry for a day or two, and then they take the bellies to the smokehouse to finish them.

(Side note for all you home curing enthusiasts . . . the vacuum machine at Swiss Meats is an actual piece of kitchen equipment invented specifically for food preparation. I don't recommend trying to fashion your own "vacuum machine" out of the Hoover in your hall closet—not only will it *not* help the seasonings to better penetrate your meat experiment but the aftermath of what it will do to your carpets might turn you off to meat forever.)

When the bacon is done drying, it goes to the Swiss Meats smokehouse, which is a pretty high-tech deal—it's a night-and-day comparison to the traditional brick smokehouses that many small-scale producers still use to this day. "The smokehouse is completely computerized and preprogrammed with a series of stages. I can be on the phone or talking to customers, or even at home mowing my grass, and this smokehouse will be doing what it's supposed to be doing." The smoke is produced by one of four different types of wood chips: hickory, maple, cherry, or apple. The chips funnel down through the device to a hot plate, and a mechanical arm goes around in a circle and scrapes off the burnt sawdust. What comes out of the three smokestacks is pure smoke. The whole process takes about eight hours. Then they cool it and start slicing.

During the slicing process, a lot of bacon ends are generated that end up going into the sausages and potato salads that are sold in the Swiss Meats retail store. They make a bacon-and-beef bratwurst that is a fantastic marriage of sausage and bacon combined into one encased package of goodness.

Once the bacon has been sliced, it is packaged using a second vacuum machine. The vacuum packaging helps the bacon to stay fresh longer. "You can keep our bacon in a refrigerator for eight weeks and in a freezer for three months. I tell everyone that if you buy a package of bacon and it's in your refrigerator for eight weeks, you shouldn't have bought it if you aren't going to eat it!" Amen to that.

BASIC BACON CURE

This easy-to-follow recipe for curing your own bacon is from Paul Brown, proprietor of the blog Mad Meat Genius (madmeatgenius.com). Paul says the secret to successfully curing bacon is balance. It's a process that is relatively simple; bacon enthusiasts should not be intimidated, regardless of your skill level in the kitchen. The key is to find the right combination of salt, sugar, and smoke. The ideal thing to do is to conduct several experiments until you discover the harmony of flavors that best appeal to your palate. Of course, that means you'll need to sample a lot of bacon in the process. How unfortunate!

8 pounds pork belly, cut into 3 or 4 sections
2 cups Morton's Sugar Cure
1 cup dark brown sugar

1. Remove the rind from the bellies using a very sharp fillet knife. If you prefer to leave the rind on, that is fine, but Paul firmly believes the rind should be removed. To do this, place the belly rind down on a cutting board. Grab the rind with a towel. With the other hand, take the knife and run it as close to the rind as possible.

2. Mix the sugar cure and brown sugar together in a bowl. Rub this mixture all over the bellies. Coat every inch of surface. Place each belly in its own heavy-duty resealable plastic bag and seal. Place the bags in the refrigerator for at least 7 days, turning them over every 2 to 3 days. You will see liquid in the bags. This is normal. It just means the process is working.

3. Place the bellies in a large pan filled with fresh water to rinse and soak them. Empty and replace the water four times over a 4-hour span. Remove the bellies and dry them off as well as you can. This is a crucial step.

4. Place the bellies on a rack with a pan underneath and let them sit in the refrigerator overnight. This process removes all moisture, so your future bacon will accept smoke. Do not worry about contamination, as the bellies are already salted and cured.

5. Now it's time to smoke the bellies. The ideal way to do this is with a smoking machine such as a Weber Smokey Mountain Smoker. If you don't have a smoker, you can improvise with your grill—just make sure that direct heat is not applied to the bellies. Choose wood chips of your preferred flavor; applewood or hickory are most commonly available at grocery stores and consistently produce a flavorful bacon. Let the bellies smoke for approximately 4 hours at 200°F. Regularly check the bellies with a thermometer to keep a close eye on their temperature. The internal temperature of the bacon should reach 150°F.

6. When the bacon is done smoking, remove it from the smoker and let it rest on a rack for 2 hours. Then your bacon is ready to cook and eat!

If for some strange reason you can't eat all 8 pounds in one sitting, wrap some in foil and store in your refrigerator or freezer for later.

CHAPTER 3

PROFILE OF A BACON NATION

HOMER SIMPSON: Are you saying you're never going to eat any animal again? What about bacon?

LISA SIMPSON: No.

HOMER: Ham?

LISA: No.

HOMER: Pork chops?

LISA: Dad, those all come from the same animal.

HOMER: Heh heh heh. Ooh, yeah, right, Lisa. A wonderful, magical animal.

A LL OF US who are united in our love of The Best Meat Ever are members of the Bacon Nation. We all pledge our allegiance to the king of meats. But even though we might be united in our passion for the mouth-watering strips of cured goodness that are produced from the underside of a pig, we must address a few important issues that threaten to divide the nation.

CIVIL WAR

While bacon lovers around the world may be united in their love for The Best Meat Ever, the Bacon Nation is divided in the debate over the best way to cook their beloved meat.

To start, you've got the Cast-Iron Skillet Mafia. They swear 100 percent by this old-school method involving a well-seasoned skillet and a stovetop or open flame. The Mafia doesn't care if bacon grease splatters all over the place. As far as they are concerned, the only way to fry bacon is by lovingly tending to it in a skillet over medium heat, turning the bacon over as many times as necessary in order to achieve the desired level of crispiness, and then draining the bacon grease into a container to save for later use. There's also no better way to distribute the scent of frying bacon throughout your dwelling than by frying it in an open cast-iron skillet. And isn't the best part of frying bacon the scent that remains in your house for hours after the meal is over? The Cast-Iron Skillet Mafia would argue yes. And if you don't agree with them, a cast-iron skillet may also double as a weapon. Consider yourself warned.

The less intimidating cousins of the Cast-Iron Skillet Mafia are the Nonstick Skillet Wannabes. These people also like frying their bacon on the stovetop, but they don't like the work involved with scrubbing the skillet clean when they're done frying the bacon. The Wannabes sometimes try to blend in with the Cast-Iron Skillet crowd to look cool, but then return to their kitchens to fry their bacon in secret with the hope that no one notices their Teflon fetish.

Betty Bakers prefer to cook their bacon in the oven. These are the neat freaks of the Bacon Nation—they're the only bacon lovers who are likely to be seen wearing an apron, and they don't even need an apron to shield themselves from bacon grease because the oven method is pretty much splatter-proof. Betty Bakers heat the oven to 350 degrees Fahrenheit, drape several slices of bacon on a rimmed baking sheet lined with aluminum foil, and bake the bacon for fifteen to twenty minutes until it has reached the perfect level of crispiness. After they move their bacon to a paper towel–lined plate to drain the excess grease, all they have to do is throw the aluminum foil in the trash and lightly scrub the baking sheet clean—all of which can be done without breaking a nail.

The Broilermakers are the rebels of the Bacon Nation. They crank up the broil setting on the oven, place a few strips of bacon on a rimmed cookie sheet, and let 'er rip. The bacon may burn before they've even had a chance to mix their first cocktail, and there's always the risk of bacon grease splattering all over the oven and igniting a grease fire. But the Broilermakers like their bacon crispy and they like it done fast. There's partying to do and the time it takes to broil bacon doesn't cramp their style.

The Nonstick Wannabes may be a bit lazy in their approach to frying bacon, and the Broilermakers may be impatient and carefree, but the Microwave Jockeys . . . well, really. They take laziness and impatience to a whole new level. The Microwave Jockeys will argue until they're blue in the face with anyone who dares to question their preferred method, swearing that microwave bacon really does taste good. But secretly they know there's nothing great about the way microwave bacon tastes—it's really just about speed and convenience. All they have to do is place a paper towel on a plate, layer it with a few slices of bacon, cover the bacon with another paper towel, and pop the plate in the microwave for about three minutes and voilà! The bacon is crispy and ready to eat, the paper towels go in the trash, and the plate goes in the dishwasher. No major cleanup is required with this method, and the bacon gets to your belly faster than through almost any other approach. The super-dedicated Microwave Jockey may even get serious and invest in a special cooking rack made specifically for microwaving bacon. With the proper equipment, Microwave Jockeys can enjoy bacon all day long while barely lifting a finger.

But as hard as it may be to believe, there is a subset of the microwave crowd that makes some Microwave Jockeys seem incredibly ambitious. I'm referring to the group of people who enjoy precooked bacon. Precooked bacon started appearing in grocery stores a few years ago. This product is exactly as it is described—the bacon has already been cooked, and it can be eaten straight out of the box or warmed in a microwave. To warm precooked bacon in the microwave takes less than a minute. I'm not kidding—in less than a minute, you can have bacon traveling down your esophagus to your stomach, barely stopping to say hi to your taste buds along the way (which in this case is usually a good thing). Precooked bacon may taste like cardboard, but it is great for those members of the Bacon Nation with attention deficit issues and a stunted sense of taste.

Traveling to the other end of the Bacon Nation spectrum, we encounter a much more ambitious group called Grill Freaks. Human evolution has happened way too quickly for this group, and the Grill Freak prefers to cook everything and anything outdoors over an open flame. This crowd contends that bacon just doesn't taste right unless it has grill marks. The dripping bacon grease may cause flames to shoot five feet into the air, but if you can't stand the heat, then step away from the grill . . . and the bacon.

Give Grill Freak a wacky redneck streak and what do you get? The Pitchfork Fondue Gourmand. The process of cooking bacon really doesn't get any more sophisticated than a vat of lard boiling over a propane-fueled flame, an event that usually takes place in a gravel or dirt parking lot. The bacon is speared onto the pitchfork, and into the vat it goes for about a minute. This gives the Gourmand just enough time to crack open a PBR (aka Pabst Blue Ribbon beer) and tell a "you might be a redneck if . . ." joke. While the time it takes to actually cook the bacon may be less than a minute, getting the lard to a boiling point takes more than an hour. But Pitchfork Fondue is an art and art can't be rushed. During that hour of standing around the vat watching the lard reach a boiling point, the seasoned Pitchfork Fondue Gourmand can polish off at least a six-pack of the aforementioned PBR. Friends should be on hand to make sure no one takes a tumble into the bubbling lard vat. That would be a most unfortunate end to what could have been a glorious day.

But lard isn't the only boiling liquid substance that can be used to cook bacon, and deep-frying isn't just an outdoor sport. If you're a professional chef with a kitchen that features a deep fryer, or if you're an enthusiastic home cook with your own personal fryer, roll some bacon around in tempura batter and throw it into a fryer full of boiling vegetable oil (or lard, if you're a hard-core purist). You can also make chicken-fried bacon using this method. Because seriously, if you're going to indulge in some bacon, then why not go all the way and have the full greasy fried experience? It's okay; no true bacon lover will judge you for your foray into true cholesterol dementia.

There's one last method that really shouldn't be mentioned due to its absurdly blasphemous nature, but no true discussion about cookin' bacon can be had without it. So this cooking method is put forth with the disclaimer that if you don't want to ruin the wonderful salty, smoky flavor of bacon, you shouldn't attempt this at all. What we're talking about here is blanching. Julia Child used to swear by this method when pork belly was needed to make a dish and the cook only had access to bacon, and the salt and smoke of bacon would overwhelm the dish. To accomplish this controversial task, you put the bacon into a saucepan of cold water, bring it to a boil, and then let it simmer for a few minutes. Blanched bacon can be useful for making French dishes such as cassoulet and coq au vin, but you won't be left with the familiar crispiness and salty taste that normally makes you so proud to be a full-fledged member of the Bacon Nation. So consider yourself warned!

Sometimes the location of your bacon cooking activities dictates which approach you prefer. Bacon fanatic Erica Whitson, who leads an online discussion about why bacon is The Best Meat Ever, used to be exclusively a pan-fryer when she lived in Southern California. But after moving to Utah, and into an apartment with a less than perfect stove, the stovetop method proved awful. It also took longer to fry the bacon because of the higher elevation. Now she is committed to baking her bacon in the oven. But she has also been known to throw a piece in the bottom of her slow cooker for bits of flavor to go with whatever she is simmering for the day. Erica is a true believer in the idea that everything should taste like bacon, no matter how you get there.

CRISPY VERSUS CHEWY

The other perennial debate among members of the Bacon Nation is over the best way to eat bacon: crispy or chewy.

We all know a member of Team Crispy. This is the person who, when ordering bacon in a restaurant, makes a very specific point of explaining to the waitress that he wants his bacon very crispy. The most obsessed fans of crispy bacon even have a specific way of describing it such as "crispy with burnt edges" or "crispy until it begins to crumble." Everyone else at the table may roll their eyes as the Crispy fanatic watches the waitress scribble the order on her notepad to ensure the message has been clearly and accurately received. But members of Team Crispy don't care—they know how they like their bacon, and anything less than charcoal is not acceptable.

People on Team Chewy aren't quite as particular. They probably won't freak out if their cheeseburger arrives topped with a crispy piece of bacon. After all, there's really no such thing as bad bacon, and they'll take it however they can get it. But when cooking bacon at home, Chewy fanatics may prefer to bake their bacon in the oven rather than frying it. As far as they are concerned, the grease and fat are just as important as the meat for the perfect bacon experience. They want it all.

However, not all bacon lovers pick a side in this battle. Some people prefer their bacon to be crispy when it's being used in a BLT or bacon cheeseburger, but they may like their bacon on the chewy side when they eat an individual slice for breakfast. To get a sense of how the Bacon Nation really feels about this vital issue, a series of surveys and man-on-the-street interviews were conducted exclusively for this book in an effort to nail down the essence of this ongoing debate. It truly is fascinating how people not only have such a strong opinion about this issue but the range of perspectives is as diverse as the Bacon Nation itself.

Chef Stefano Frigerio of Mio Restaurant in Washington, DC, prefers his bacon crispy. "My wife loves it crispy, and she's usually the one cooking breakfast! But I actually like it crispy—I don't like it when it's too chewy."

David Lebovitz, a chef and author currently living in Paris, also decidedly prefers his bacon crispy. "Soggy bacon is awful. What's the point?"

Ronny Drennan of Broadbent Hams in western Kentucky likes his bacon crispy, as long as it's not overcooked. "People cook it too fast. If you cook it wrong, you can make it so hard you can hardly bite through it."

Brooks Reynolds of Des Moines, Iowa, sits squarely in the middle on this issue. And he even uses steak terms to describe his favorite way for bacon to be cooked, "I like my bacon medium rare! Crispy on the outer edges but nice and chewy in the center."

June Scott of Scott Hams in Kentucky likes her bacon chewy, and she likes to cook it on her George Foreman grill. "With the George Foreman grill, you don't have to cut the rind off because it will hold it down. It's real easy. In about only five minutes it's done but still chewy and in six minutes it's crispy."

Moving to the extreme chewy end of the spectrum we have Jason Lewis, owner of a company called Lollyphile that produces maple bacon–flavored lollipops. Jason prefers it "as close to raw as I can get before I start to worry about getting sick (which hasn't ever happened). If I get really expensive bacon from a specialty store, I'll just warm it up a little." Jason isn't the only one who likes his bacon rare. Chef Todd Gray of the restaurant Equinox in Washington, DC, also likes his bacon on the oink side. "I prefer my bacon chewy. My brother and I used to eat it raw when we were children, right out of the fridge."

No matter where you stand in this debate, we can all agree that Bacon is The Best Meat Ever, whichever way it's prepared.

PIG IN A POKE: BACON REMEDIES

Should you decide that your love of bacon needs to extend to your basic medical care, you might consider engaging in any combination of the following activities:

- SPLINTERS. If you get a splinter, wrap a strip of bacon around the area where the splinter went in. The grease from the bacon will eventually help the splinter slide out.

- WARTS. Raw bacon is one of the many home remedies supposedly used as a cure for the annoying problem of warts or verrucas. Apply a strip to the offending bump and wait for the magic to happen.

- BOILS. Apply fat from bacon to the boil and let sit ten to fifteen minutes per day. The boil will come to a head in three to ten days and will drain on its own. This seems to defy common sense, but some swear by it.

- COMMON COLD. At the first sign of a cold, make a "bacon plaster" to wear day and night. To make the plaster, take a slice of fatty bacon, place between two pieces of muslin or cheesecloth, and attach it to the chest with tape. You may pass out from the smell, which can be potent, but the bacon keeps the chest clear and wards off congestion.

- POISONOUS BITES. This particular remedy is truly bizarre, but again, some swear by it: if you're bitten and the area turns beet red and/or black, seek medical help, but also buy a pound of bacon and wrap the entire area with many strips. Leave the bacon in place overnight and by the next morning upon awakening, you will see most if not all of the infection gone and your regular skin color. The bacon will be "cooked" from the infection, but don't eat it. (Really? That ruins my breakfast plans.) If you have some persistent redness, do it again the following night. And don't forget to hit the emergency room!

CELEBRATING BACON

Putting differences aside, members of the Bacon Nation from around the world often come together to celebrate our beloved meat.

The Blue Ribbon Bacon Festival in Des Moines, Iowa, is a newly formed but up-and-coming tribute to The Best Meat Ever. Appropriately located in the Pork Capital of America, this annual event attracts a devoted group of bacon lovers for a day of festivities that culminates in a bacon-eating contest. And of course there is an abundant supply of bacon-blessed foods available to participants throughout the day, along with a plentiful supply of alcohol to keep the spirited masses happy. The next day you may not remember how much bacon you consumed at the event, but you'll have a good time there no matter what because it's truly all about the bacon.

Des Moines is also the host city of the annual World Pork Expo. This industry-focused event at the Iowa State Fairgrounds is devoted to all things porcine. As you walk down the midway toward the various exhibition buildings, the scent of barbecuing pork products permeates the air and is almost more than any rational bacon-loving person can handle. Even worse (or better, depending on how you look at it), many of the food samples are free. Yes, you read that correctly—for a small admission fee, you get all the free pork products you can consume in a day. Why more people haven't caught on to this amazing little secret about the World Pork Expo and doubled the size of its attendance is beyond me. The temptations at this event are numerous, thrilling, and a serious threat to one's waistline.

Living History Farms just outside of Des Moines is dedicated to educating people about the history of Iowa, including the growth of its famous pork industry. The museum often conducts workshops and events on topics ranging from the history of curing bacon to building the perfect BLT. It's a genuine opportunity to connect with your deeply felt love of bacon and to learn wonderful new ways to apply it.

While they may pale in comparison to Iowa's status as the heart of the Bacon Nation, several other states also host their own annual bacon-focused events. Bacon and Beans Days in Augusta, Wisconsin, takes place around the Fourth of July holiday and is an opportunity to simultaneously pledge your allegiance to both the United States of America and the Bacon Nation while gobbling up your favorite pork product. For the members of the Bacon Nation, eating the beans is optional.

Since the late 1960s, the Preble County Pork Festival in Eaton, Ohio, has taken place every year during the third week in September. Bacon is just one of dozens of pork products featured at this widely attended and wildly popular event. You can even learn how to butcher and prepare your own pork products. And the pig races are always a highlight! The Tipton County Pork Festival in Tipton, Indiana, also celebrates the hog, country style. Since 1969, Indiana members of the Bacon Nation have been flocking to this event, also held in early September.

Not to be outdone by all of those pesky midwestern pork-producing states, the Virginia Pork Festival in Greensville County serves more than 43,000 pounds of pork per year at this annual event. The event is so popular that it is limited to 15,000 attendees per year. The list of pork products you can indulge in is quite extensive, but those who are bacon focused can enjoy a good ol' BLT, among other things.

Just in case you've been laboring under the delusion that the Bacon Nation stops at the U.S. borders, think again. It is a global community, and events celebrating various forms of cured pork products can be found in many other countries. The Gailtaler Speckfest in Hermagor, Austria, features plenty of food, beer, and entertainment to "get your pork on" in this small town near the border with Italy. Another European event is the Foire au Lard (Bacon Fair) that has been taking place in Martigny, Switzerland, since the 1800s. Like manna from heaven, farmers from the region descend upon the center of town to sell their bacon, sausages, ham, and cheese to the general public.

All of these annual events around the world are fabulous, but nothing can possibly compete with the Chinese Year of the Pig as a celebration of all things porcine. An entire year dedicated to celebrating the pig—it's like 365 days of Christmas! Unfortunately it only happens every twelve years, but there's no question it's worth the wait and you've got eleven years in between each celebration to properly plan and prepare. Beyond being the most delicious animal of the entire Chinese zodiac, in Chinese culture one of the things pigs represent is fertility. So for an entire year you not only have a reason to consume bacon with wild abandon but tradition also implies that you should alternate your pork-eating sessions with procreation-oriented activities. Seriously, people, given this yearlong mandate of Sex and Bacon (which, by the way, is the title of a really entertaining book by Sarah Katherine Lewis), how can the pig *not* be the most wonderful, magical animal ever, and how can bacon *not* be The Best Meat Ever? It really is great to be a member of the Bacon Nation.

SECRET BACON BEHAVIOR

Devoted members of the Bacon Nation don't need an organized event to indulge in copious amounts of bacon on a regular basis. For some bacon enthusiasts, all it takes is a trip to their local bacon-friendly dining establishment for a personal bacon celebration.

Jason Mosley, who is also known as Mr. Baconpants and has a blog of the same name, likes to eat bacon at a place called Fat Heads in Pittsburgh's South Side. "They have a great selection of beer and their food is out of this world. I usually get the bacon cheeseburger, which is about the size of my head. It's loaded with mayo, lettuce, a thick slice of tomato, and four rashers of crispy bacon. If I am really in the bacon mood I will also get an order of bacon cheese fries. There is nothing better than drinking an IPA beer and munching on a bacon cheese-burger."

Mr. Baconpants also likes to take his bacon festivities on the road. "My most memorable story involving bacon is the time I got the ultimate bacon cheeseburger in Las Vegas. In the Mirage Hotel there is a restaurant called the Burger Bar. They give you choices of meat, bun, and toppings. On the list of toppings were four different kinds of bacon: applewood, pepper, cinnamon, and jalapeño. So I got all four kinds (sixteen strips of bacon) on a burger with provolone cheese. The waiter gave me a funny look. Let me just say it was amazing; with every bite I got a taste of something different. I will never forget that burger."

Steph, one of the readers of your faithful author's blog Bacon Unwrapped, decided to get together with co-workers and make bacon candy after crunching some numbers and determining it would be cheaper to make their own than to order bacon chocolate candy from Vosges Haut-Chocolat. "My co-workers and I are a bit bacon obsessed. When we calculated how much it would cost to have a single pound of Vosges Flying Chocolate Pigs shipped to us, we choked. I quipped, 'Get me a pig form and I'll make you chocolate pigs!' Two weeks later, pig candy molds arrived in the mail. We've been happily experimenting with the various forms of chocolate and various flavors of bacon ever since. We grill the bacon first for an added smoky depth to the final candy."

Another Bacon Unwrapped reader, Michelle Stokes, also chooses to celebrate bacon with co-workers. "My company has quarterly meetings in the early morning where bacon is provided with breakfast. My team had a bacon-eating contest one morning. I took the title by putting away sixty strips of bacon. My only real competition put away fifty-six strips." That's one aggressive (and very impressive) start to the workday.

And last but not least, Bacon Unwrapped reader Velma takes her bacon celebration much more seriously. At her family's Thanksgiving event, one of the things they are thankful for is a plentiful stash of bacon. "To celebrate Thanksgiving we have an annual 'Bacon Fest.' While the parade is on, we cook many, many pounds of bacon. Bacon is then added to *every* dish on the table: the turkey is basted with bacon fat, crumbled bacon is added to the sweet spuds, mashed potatoes, stuffing, broccoli, and yes, even the pumpkin pie. There's something about the threat of a coronary that introduces an element of danger to our elegant table."

So whether they're celebrating their love of bacon by eating it while downing steins of beer in the Alps, inhaling it by the platter at a family reunion, or scarfing it down in the semiprivacy of their cubicle at work, citizens of the Bacon Nation will stop at nothing to get as much of their beloved meat as possible. Bless their little cholesterol-clogged hearts.

CHAPTER 4

BACON OR FAKIN'?

"I really like bacon. I was vegetarian for a year
and then I smelled a bacon sandwich at an airport and said
'screw this.'"
—Craig Ferguson

THERE IS A big elephant in the room that threatens to trample the theory that bacon is The Best Meat Ever. The issue is that a significant part of the world's population does not eat bacon. As hard as this may be for the most zealous members of the Bacon Nation to understand, it must be discussed before we go any further.

The most obvious and understandable non–bacon eating part of this crowd are those who don't eat it for religious reasons. Many people who are of Jewish or Islamic faith do not consume pork in any form, let alone bacon.

It is worth mentioning that this author has friends who were raised in a conservative Jewish, bacon-free environment. But whether as a result of their friendship with the author or other outside influences over the years, those previously observant Jews now secretly indulge in bacon on a regular basis. Even the deepest religious beliefs can't keep some people away from The Best Meat Ever.

Why does Judaism frown upon consumption of the pork? Theories abound, but the most commonly accepted reason stems from the Old Testament. According to Leviticus,

> *and the swine, though he divide the hoof, and be cloven footed, yet he cheweth not the cud; he is unclean to you. Of their flesh shall ye not eat, and their carcass shall ye not touch, they are unclean to you.*

Or in lay terms, according to the Bible animals are only kosher if they both chew their cud and have split hooves. Pigs have split hooves but do not chew their cud, hence making them technically not kosher. There you have it.

Islam also frowns upon the consumption of pork, except in cases when it must be consumed to avoid starvation. This is a practice that stems from passages in their holy book, the Q'uran, forbidding the handling or consumption of swine.

Even if you don't share these religious beliefs, everyone has a right to believe and practice as they choose. So let us withhold judgment for the next topic . . . vegetarians.

VEGETARIANS: THE OTHER, OTHER WHITE MEAT

Vegetarians are a mysterious bunch. It's understandable that some people can't eat certain foods for health or religious reasons, but why someone would voluntarily choose to give up an entire food category—a food category that, let's be serious, is a large reason why humans are at the top of the food chain—is incredibly difficult for those of us who worship at the House of Bacon to understand. It just doesn't seem to make any sense.

However, as previously mentioned, everyone has the right to live how they choose to live. So we'll leave it at that. For now.

The vegetarian population seems to be growing as evidenced by the increasing number of retail options dedicated to the lifestyle. There are also thousands of vegetarian bloggers who share recipes and information about their lifestyle online daily. Clearly, vegetarianism is here to stay. However, a recent strain of vegetarianism has emerged that is willing to admit that the hardest thing about giving up meat is, not surprisingly, bacon. As difficult as it may be for bacon lovers to understand vegetarianism, a certain segment of the vegetarian population may actually help prove the point that bacon is The Best Meat Ever by admitting it is the meat they miss the most. Why else would they create a product out of tofu that is meant to taste like bacon? So I guess those crazy vegetarians deserve a little credit!

THE BIG BACON TENT

Whether inspired by religious or dietary circumstances, or out of a general desire to make more food taste like bacon (and understandably so), today an entire industry exists for the purpose of producing nonpork products that theoretically create the same sensations one experiences when eating pork bacon.

The debate about whether or not these products can really be called bacon can get quite intense. Some people consider the use of the word "bacon" to describe nonpork products to be blasphemous. Others think that imitation is the most sincere form of flattery and therefore have no problem with nonpork products aspiring to bacon's status as The Best Meat Ever (even though they know that anything other than pork bacon will never reach the top). What we can do is present some facts so you can make up your own mind and be armed with the information you need to argue your side of this important issue the next time you encounter someone who wants to "take it outside."

Let's start by taking a look at the definition of the word "bacon" according to a few different sources.

Dictionary.com defines bacon as "the back and sides of the hog, salted and dried or smoked, usually sliced thin and fried for food." Nothing to protest there—we can all agree with that assessment. *The American Heritage Dictionary* defines it as "the salted and smoked meat from the back and sides of a pig." Now we're starting to build some consensus. *Merriam-Webster's Online Dictionary* defines it as "a side of a pig cured and smoked." Need we really say more? According to these widely respected sources, there is no question that bacon is meant to describe a cured meat product derived from the central regions of a pig.

The only source that takes some liberties with the definition of bacon is Wiktionary. There, bacon is described as "a cut of meat from the sides, belly, or back of a pig, particularly, or sometimes other animals." Even though Wiktionary acknowledges that bacon may come from critters other than pigs, they still define bacon as coming from the sides, belly, or back of those other animals. So even if bacon isn't all about the pig, it's definitely all about an animal's midsection (not to mention the impact bacon sometimes has on the midsection of its consumers).

With these definitions in mind, let's take a look at a few nonpork products that are called bacon. The first nonpork bacon that most people are familiar with is turkey bacon. Those who prefer to eat turkey bacon instead of pork bacon probably make this choice largely for health reasons. And for our observant Jewish friends, it's the closest they can get to tasting the real thing without crossing the line. So that's all good and fair. But even if you define bacon as Wiktionary does, and allow for bacon to come from an animal other than a pig, turkey bacon doesn't technically come from the "sides, belly, or back" of a turkey. It is a processed version of turkey meat—most likely breast—that is then smoked to taste like bacon. That's a major strike against it. Next to tofu bacon, which we'll get to later on, turkey bacon is probably the most processed, artificial form of bacon available on the market. Yet turkey bacon has been produced by companies such as Butterball and Louis Rich for many years, and it is a very popular product. So if you love turkey bacon and want to insist on its legitimate bacon status, its mere longevity as a food product is on your side of the argument. It still doesn't change the fact that if you held a strip of pork bacon next to a strip of turkey bacon, it's pretty difficult to find any similarities between the two meats. As far as bacon fanatics are concerned, it's impossible for turkey bacon to compete with a crispy strip of pork bacon; the two are in very different leagues.

Turkeys aren't the only bird trying to get in on some bacon action. Duck bacon is another product that can be found at specialty grocery stores and through independent producers. D'Artagnan makes a popular version that is nitrate and nitrite free. As with turkey bacon, duck bacon is merely a slice of duck meat smoked to resemble the taste of bacon. But the only thing about it that resembles bacon is that it has a smoky flavor and comes in strips. It is also sliced incredibly thin and takes only about ten seconds to fry before it shrivels up completely, which is a fascinating event to observe.

Another form of nonpork bacon that is gaining in popularity is beef bacon. If you like beef and you enjoy really salty foods, then beef bacon is for you! There is nothing happier than pork and beef bacon living side by side in harmony at Christmas morning breakfast. Just be careful, because you might wake up one day to find that you crave the saltiness of the beef bacon more than pork bacon. Although unlikely to happen, it is a thought to keep in mind. Consider yourself warned.

While a couple of the major bacon companies produce a prepackaged beef bacon product (the most notable being the Smithfield version produced under the Gwaltney brand name), beef bacon isn't as commonly available in grocery stores the same way that turkey bacon is. Most people get their beef bacon from a specialty butcher. Beef bacon is usually made by curing and smoking a brisket, which comes from the breast of a cow. Well, at least beef bacon comes from an area of the cow that is close to the belly!

Lamb bacon is the nonpork bacon product that comes closest to meeting the technical definition of bacon. Lamb bacon is actually made from the belly of a lamb. Chef Ethan McKee is one chef who has experimented with using lamb bellies to make bacon. The result is a surprising culinary delight. He first began to experiment with lamb bacon as chef de cuisine at the highly acclaimed restaurant Equinox in Washington, DC.

Chef McKee (who is now the executive chef of another restaurant in northwest DC called Rock Creek) first experimented with lamb bacon because he hated to see lamb bellies go to waste. "At the time I started experimenting with lamb bacon at Equinox, we had a saddle of lamb on the menu, which was the loin of a lamb. The way it came to us from the meat company, the belly was still connected to the loin. We had these pieces of lamb belly that we weren't using, and it was just bugging me that we weren't really doing anything with it. So I decided to experiment with making lamb bacon. It's the exact same process to cure lamb belly as it is to cure pork belly and you can flavor it however you want with different spices."

Like many chefs around the world, as well as home cooks who enjoy the process of curing their own meats, Chef McKee learned most of what he knows by buying a bunch of books and experimenting— classic trial and error. "From culinary school, I knew a few basic rules, but there's nothing really too tough about it. Most charcuterie is really measured recipes—there's a ratio of salt to meat, and once you have that down you can do whatever you want with other seasonings and flavorings. But it's something I love to do. It's a very satisfying thing to do." And the resulting product is equally satisfying for bacon lovers.

Even though the lamb bacon experiment turned out well, it never quite made it onto the Equinox menu. Rather, it was reserved for VIP customers—people who are real food enthusiasts who would be into trying something as unexpected as lamb bacon. "You'd have to be pretty into food to appreciate something like that. If most people saw lamb belly on the menu, they'd wonder what the hell it is. But people who are foodies and who are into that kind of thing think it's really cool."

If lamb bacon is the nonpork bacon most similar to the real thing, then tofu bacon is at the opposite end of the spectrum. This product is also sometimes called veggie bacon or fakin' bacon, and it is the ideal product for the vegetarian who simply can't quit bacon, but who doesn't miss it enough to cross back over to the meat side. Tofu bacon is usually made with some combination of tofu, liquid smoke, salt, and soy sauce. A company called LightLife makes a tofu bacon they call Smart Bacon that is sold through select retail stores.

Kathleen Evey Walters, of Washington, DC, is a vegetarian who cooks with tofu bacon but accepts its limitations. "I am not a huge fan of it in its pure form, i.e., eaten alone as bacon. However, I made a great breakfast casserole once for a work event using fakin' bacon, and honestly, *no one* knew it wasn't real bacon until I told them! As strips of bacon alone, however, it does not match up to the real thing . . . there's more to eating than flavor."

Given that tofu doesn't come from an animal, this product really doesn't stand up to the "is it bacon?" test. But if it helps a vegetarian get through the day, and if it's good enough for use in certain dishes to the point that nonvegetarians don't even notice the difference, then it could be said that tofu bacon is serving an important role in modern-day society.

Since all nonpork bacon products claim to be a healthier alternative to pork bacon, and since pork bacon is constantly defending itself against the argument that it is a threat to the well-being of humankind, I thought we should take a look at some cold, hard facts about all of the bacon products out there. Duck bacon and lamb bacon aren't quite as mainstream, so we'll leave them out of the study for now. This comparison will take a look at turkey bacon, beef bacon, tofu bacon, and pork bacon.

Type of Bacon (based on a 14 g serving)	Overall Calories	Calories from Fat	Total Amount of Fat	Cholesterol	Sodium
Tofu (LightLife Smart Bacon)	26	NA	1 g	0 mg	198 mg
Turkey (Louis Rich)	35	25	2.5 g	15 mg	180 mg
Beef (Gwaltney)	46	37	4 g	10 mg	123 mg
Pork (Oscar Mayer Naturally Hardwood Smoked)	70	50	6 g	15 mg	290 mg

SOURCES: HTTP://WWW.FOODFACTS.COM/ AND HTTP://WWW.LIGHTLIFE.COM, ACCESSED 8/1/08

SWINE GEOGRAPHY

According to MapQuest, the following states have a place or town called Bacon: Idaho, Indiana, Missouri, Ohio, Texas, and Washington. And there is even a Bacon County in Georgia. What a delicious road trip that would be!

• The nickname for Cincinnati is **Porkopolis**, which dates back to the early 1800s when Cincinnati was a major hog-packing center for the United States, and it wasn't unusual to see hogs roaming the streets of town.

• The Baltimore neighborhood called **Pigtown** isn't just a place to find a good BLT. This neighborhood got its name because it is where the railroad used to drop off pigs that were then herded through the streets to slaughterhouses.

• You might be able to find some good ribs in **Hog Back**, Kansas. And you can pick up some pork jowl bacon in the town of **Hog Jaw** in Alabama or Arkansas. Last, you can work off the calories from your bacon road trip with a hike around **Hog Mountain**, Georgia.

Now you have the facts and can make an informed decision. True, classic bacon is the most caloric, but is it intrinsically really all that bad? And let's not forget that taste and sheer enjoyment need to be taken into consideration. But as in all things, consume bacon in moderation—whether your obsession is tofu bacon or the kind that comes from the wonderful, magical animal that is the pig.

SHOULD *EVERYTHING* TASTE LIKE BACON?

In addition to imitation bacon products, there are also several bacon-flavored condiment options available to give consumers the ability to make everything they eat taste like bacon. Because who in their right mind wouldn't want that?

McCormick's Bac'n Pieces and Betty Crocker Bac-Os have been providing instant gratification to bacon lovers for generations. Like tofu bacon, these products get their bacony flavor from soy products and smoke flavoring. Regardless of whether or not you think these products actually taste like bacon, you can't deny that there's something appealing about the idea of having bacon at your fingertips 24/7.

A company called Flavor Spray is now selling a liquid product called Smoked Bacon Spray. With just a couple of spritzes, you can give any food a smoky taste resembling bacon. This stuff is pretty intense, and it tastes more like smoke than like bacon, but again—instant gratification is the name of the game (just don't spray it directly on your tongue if you want to be able to taste anything else ever again).

Finally, there is a curiously appealing product called Bacon Salt that first appeared on the market in 2007. This product has gained quickly in popularity partially due to the creative marketing efforts of the inventors of Bacon Salt, Justin and Dave. But Bacon Salt owes most of its success to the fact that it really does taste like bacon. Of all the nonpork bacon products that have been invented over the last several decades, Bacon Salt is easily the most realistic product to date. And good news for all of those people who can't eat bacon for religious or dietary reasons—miraculously, there is not a single ounce of pork in Bacon Salt. It is 100 percent kosher. Bacon Salt comes in a few flavors, including original, hickory, and pepper.

Given that Bacon Salt is kosher, the story behind its creation is quite humorous. Bacon Salt cofounder Justin came up with the idea for Bacon Salt while at a Jewish military wedding as he espoused the virtues of bacon and a drink called a Mitch Morgan (a shot of bourbon with a bacon garnish) to a table full of people who kept kosher. When he told this story to his friend Dave, the other eventual cofounder of Bacon Salt, they both knew what they had to do and they set out on a mission to make everything taste like bacon. And regardless of whether you like or dislike the concept of bacon substitutes, that notion that everything should taste like bacon should be supported wholeheartedly by every member of the Bacon Nation.

PART II

THE BACON DIET

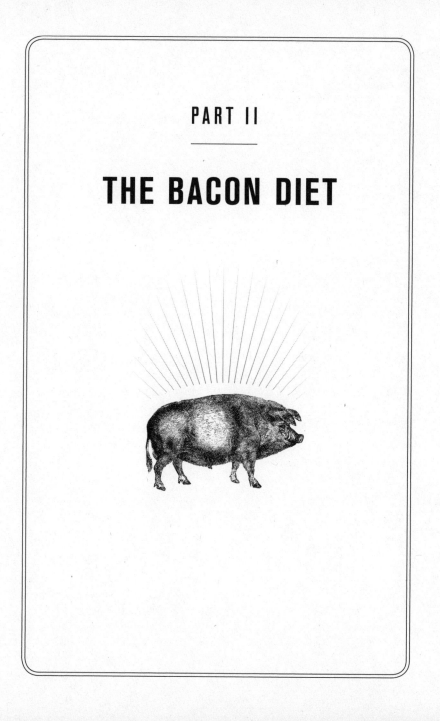

CHAPTER 5

THE CULINARY AND CULTURAL
RENAISSANCE OF BACON

"We are living in the Golden Age of Bacon."
—Bill Marvel, *The Dallas Morning News*,
December 13, 2006

IT SEEMS AS if everyone is talking about bacon these days. It's showing up at an increasing number of restaurants around the country, and more consumers are seeking out specialty bacons over the Internet and at local farmers' markets. There's an ongoing quest to find the best version of The Best Meat Ever.

THE RISE OF THE BACON BLOG

The trend toward openly expressing one's love for bacon in a public forum has led to a number of blogs on the topic. Prior to the launch of Bacon Unwrapped in June 2005, a few other bacon lovers had already begun to blaze the bacon blogging trail. I ❤ Bacon (iheartbacon.com) was the most popular bacon blog at the time in terms of readership, and even though its author stopped updating her blog regularly in the summer of 2007, her pioneering bacon blogging efforts are still a popular source for bacon-obsessed browsers of the Web. In the last two years, several other bacon blogs have come and gone, and as of mid-2008 there were about a dozen regular bloggers using the word "bacon" in their titles and writing about the topic at least a couple of times per month, if not several times per week. Beyond bacon-specific bloggers, countless other food bloggers are also including bacon in their daily adventures in the kitchen. So in the same way that the popularity of bacon as a food product continues to increase over time, its presence online is expanding.

Another bacon blog started in 2005 and still thriving is The Bacon Show (baconshow.blogspot.com). The mysterious mastermind behind this blog launched his love poem to bacon with the singular goal of posting "one bacon recipe per day, every day, forever." So far, The Bacon Show has lived up to that promise. It makes most other bacon blogging efforts look half-assed. As this book went to press, well over

1,000 bacon recipes have been posted on the site sourced from cookbooks, Web sites, restaurants, newspapers, and bacon fanatics. The recipes range from everyday dishes like buttermilk cornbread with bacon to more exotic fare like wild game jambalaya with alligator tail, wild boar bacon, and kangaroo sausage. And who wouldn't want that for Sunday supper?

The creator and author of The Bacon Show prefers to remain anonymous, so he shall be referred to here as TBS. When asked how the idea for The Bacon Show came about, TBS provided a response that is far more philosophical than one might expect from someone whose sole mission is to simply publish one bacon recipe per day: "The Bacon Show started as a double desire to give voice to an obsession and to fill a perceived lack. The obsession was, of course, bacon; the perceived lack was an environment in which the obsession could converse and function." Obsession really seems to be a constant theme with the Bacon Nation. More plainly, The Bacon Show started as a conversation between TBS and a friend. "We were both producing bacon-related artwork at the time—I was engaged in a week-long diet strictly of bacon, taking photographs and writing poems, and my friend was working on a series of large-format drawings of bacon—and thought that it would be fun to exhibit the work and serve bacon at the opening. We eventually thought it would be more engaging if we invited other artists to participate. And so, the real Bacon Show started as a multimedia exhibition in an empty apartment in Brooklyn, New York, featuring the work of twenty or so artists, musicians, and writers. The environment that we aimed to create was, at least, partially achieved; there was conversation and function both." A celebration of bacon was born.

No one has embraced the concept of bacon as an art form as much as TBS. With bacon as the source of inspiration, The Bacon Show naturally evolved over time. "The Bacon Show exhibition ran for two consecutive years, and eventually turned into an annual Bacon Party, in which every attendee had to bring a dish featuring bacon in some innovative way: cartoons and early episodes of Julia Child's *The French Chef* were projected on the walls; audio recordings were made of people reminiscing about bacon; a book of bacon-related poems and quotations was distributed, along with buttons, refrigerator magnets, and so on." Once the bacon train starts rolling down the tracks, there really is no stopping it.

"Simultaneous to this was the idea that there was a whole universe of bacon and bacon-related recipes out there. My sister had given me a copy of Sara Perry's beautifully compiled *Everything Tastes Better with Bacon*, and I began thinking to myself, what if someone went a step further, and instead of compiling a selection of recipes, compiled the entirety of all known bacon recipes, in a set of encyclopedia volumes, meticulously arranged and cross-referenced. I still dream about this, and the challenge has been set. I don't care if it is me or someone else, I would love it to exist either way. The Bacon Show blog grew out of that idea, though in a toned-down, modest format. After all, you have to start somewhere."

And to think some people start a blog because one night they find themselves in a situation where they've had one too many cocktails and easy access to a computer. It's good to know that someone takes his craft seriously.

Finding one new bacon recipe per day seems like an exercise that would be quite challenging, but not so according to TBS. "Bacon recipes are everywhere, and though many overlap in major or minor ways, there are still enough to satisfy an entire life, without repetition. The Internet is, obviously, a thrillingly comprehensive sea of information, and the community of food bloggers and critics is an incredibly active wave within that. I consult magazines, cookbooks, organic farming brochures and catalogs, the sides of food packaging, tattered and greasy index cards buried on the bottom shelves of pantries. If someone prepares a dish I have never encountered before, I have them write the recipe out." Bacon recipes seem to come crawling out of the woodwork in droves for an appearance on The Bacon Show.

It still is hard to believe that it is so easy to find a new bacon recipe every day. But TBS seems to have no problem finding daily bacon inspiration. "I am constantly surprised at how many recipes there actually are, and how if there were ever a print volume collection of these recipes, it would require its own zoning permits. To be honest, also: if I am ever stumped, it is usually because I am searching for recipes early in the morning, when my brain has not yet fully grown into the day. Again, there are bacon recipes everywhere, which attests to the love with which bacon is upheld and possessed. Love will test one's innovation, to constantly stay a step ahead of the antagonists that come preying after it." How poetic and practical.

HAMMY HUMOR

David Sutherland may be one of the biggest bacon enthusiasts of all time. From 1984 through 1988, he drew the comic book *The Beano*, which featured Dennis the Menace's pet pig Rasher. The strip also featured Rasher's family, including his brother Hamlet, his sister Virginia Ham, Uncle Crackling, and Little Piglet.

BACON IN THE ZEITGEIST

The online dialogue about bacon isn't limited just to blogs like The Bacon Show. Numerous discussion boards around the Internet are dedicated to the topic. On food enthusiast Web sites with active discussion boards, conversations are regularly launched about bacon in which users discuss topics ranging from the best place to find bacon in a particular city to an exchange of opinions about specific brands of bacon. One such online discussion about bacon is on a Web site called Lounge of Tomorrow. On January 9, 2007, Erica Whitson, who is known on the site as blueerica, posted an item suggesting that "bacon is meat candy" and encouraging the community to discuss. The response was overwhelming. As of October 2008, twenty-two months after the discussion was launched, the Lounge of Tomorrow bacon discussion thread was still alive and thriving. More than a thousand comments have been contributed to the conversation, mostly in the form of various personal tributes to everyone's favorite meat.

The saying "Bacon is Meat Candy" actually emerged from an unexpected source a couple of years ago, as often happens with anything to do with bacon, given its universal appeal. The source of this phrase was a daily sports show on ESPN called *Around the Horn*. The format is a rapid-fire roundtable discussion about sports issues of the day between the host, Tony Reali, and four sports reporters from around the country. Woody Paige, a sportswriter for *The Denver Post*, is a regular on the show and an incredibly amusing character. Woody always has a chalkboard behind his head, and throughout the show he displays witty, humorous proverbs that rarely have anything to do with the sports topic at hand, but are entertaining nonetheless. One day a couple of years ago, "Bacon is Meat Candy" was Woody's idiomatic gem during one of the show's segments. Erica caught it, memorialized it on Lounge of Tomorrow, and the rest is history.

The Lounge of Tomorrow gang isn't just a group of cyber friends—they actually get together in person regularly to celebrate their love of bacon. Erica recently moved from California to Utah, and at her going-away party she was showered with dozens of bacon-inspired gifts ranging from bacon-flavored toothpicks to Bacon Salt. Bacon has become a way of bonding for this group of friends, and Erica thinks it's "cool what bacon has come to mean for us as a group, and for me personally. I smell bacon, hear a sizzle, find it on a burger or as a topping, and I think of my friends." Lounge of Tomorrow creator Steve Zlick adds that "bacon is not only delicious, it has become almost synonymous with 'cool' or 'swanky' among our crowd . . . as in, 'he's so bacon' or 'that's totally bacon!'" The Lounge of Tomorrow group is a fine example of the power bacon has to unite people everywhere.

While the Lounge of Tomorrow group uses bacon to describe someone's cool factor, others use bacon to describe their perfect mate. In an interview for an article in *dsm Magazine*'s annual "Men's Book," one man shared his idea of the perfect woman:

> *I describe the perfect woman like I describe a perfect piece of bacon. They have a lot in common. They're sweet, good looking, full of character, and not too abrasive but bold and confident, preferably Iowa raised. Not too thin, but not too thick. . . . She comes from good stock. She's the real deal—not of the vegetarian variety.*

Bacon as an analogy for the ideal woman? If that doesn't demonstrate the power of bacon, I don't know what does.

BACON LOVE SONGS

In the same way that there are bloggers who write daily love poems to bacon, you'd be surprised by the number of musical artists who have written songs about their favorite meat.

The bluegrass country band Chatham County Line sings a song titled "Bacon in the Skillet." Their lyrics are an uncomplicated tribute to The Best Meat Ever:

> *Sometimes I get so hungry I'd eat it up right off the floor.*
> *There's bacon in the skillet, sweet taters in the pan.*

What a sweet lullaby to sing yourself to sleep with.

Roger Alan Wade is another country artist with a bacon fetish. His song "Fryin' Bacon Nekkid" is a classic song of heartbreak that uses bacon as an analogy for his pain.

> *Lovin' you is like fryin' bacon nekkid.*
> *You tempt me darling, and then you torture me.*

(WARNING: Unless you have a splatter-proof method, this author advises you *not* to attempt "fryin' bacon nekkid" at home.)

Bacon seems to be quite popular with country music artists. Craig Morgan also mentions bacon in his hit song "Little Bit of Life" when he lists bacon as one of the simple pleasures in life:

> *A little bit of bacon.*
> *. . . A little bit of life.*

A "whole lot of bacon" would be much better than a little bit of bacon but we can all agree that bacon is definitely the key to a happy life.

ShitKickers are a country band with a more irreverent approach to their music, but who are equally devoted to bacon. Their song "Bacon" is only thirty-eight seconds long, but it succinctly depicts how many of us feel about bacon, and the pain that is felt when bacon can't be found. Their desire can be summed up by this one line from the song: "All I want is a big ol' plate of bacon." ShitKickers' other song devoted to bacon, "Beer 'n' Bacon," talks about waking up to bacon in the morning:

> Beer and bacon waitin' for my friends.
> They ain't comin' over, but I'm not staying sober.

Who needs friends anyway when you've got bacon and beer for breakfast?

Country artists aren't the only ones singing about our favorite meat. The Canadian rock band Screamin' Rico and the Canadian Back Bacon Boys make it pretty clear how they feel about their beloved meat just by the name of their band. And their album Sex, Bacon and Rock and Roll is a comedic journey that contains a track simply called "Bacon." The song offers some simple advice:

> Bacon, lettuce and tomato. . . .
> Try it with some mayo . . .
> Fry it up, put the oil in a cup. Bacon.

Thus proving that music doesn't need to be complicated to be entertaining or inspirational.

Everyone's favorite rapper, Snoop Dogg, also mentions bacon in one of his songs. In the song "Pimp Slapp'd," an attack on the questionable behavior of others in the rap industry, Snoop proclaims his music to be the best with "so put the bacon in the skillet, and try to peel it, cause Doggystyle Records is the realest." Who really knows what those lyrics really mean, but what we do know is that bacon is tha B-to-tha-izzest mizzle killa fo sho.

Snoop Dogg is pretty hard to top, but there is another bacon-loving band whose antics reign supreme. Any true child of the eighties has a special place in their heart for the hard-rock band Metallica. So when it was recently revealed that one of Metallica's backstage demands is "bacon, very important that bacon be available at every meal and during the day," the Bacon Nation's respect for the band rose to a whole new level. Eating bacon backstage with Metallica would seriously be the coolest thing ever.

BACONSUMERISM

Why should bacon lovers around the world draw the line at simply eating the stuff? Here are just a few of the bacon-themed products on the market today:

- **Bacon strip bandages** (bacon cures all)
- **Bacon lunch boxes** (perfect for transporting a BLT)
- **Bacon wallets** (perfect for transporting money to buy more bacon)
- **Bacon-flavored toothpicks** (freshen up your bacon breath after dinner)
- **Bacon wristbands** (so you remember to bring home some bacon)
- **Bacon scarves** (even people are better when they are wrapped in bacon)
- **Bacon Christmas ornaments** (bacon is delicious *and* festive)
- **Bacon chocolate bars** (don't knock it until you try it!)

FROM GREASY SPOON TO SILVER SPOON: BACON AND THE CHEFS WHO LOVE IT

Bacon has always had a presence in restaurants with a casual dining environment. Practically every diner on the face of the planet features bacon for breakfast, BLTs for lunch, and bacon cheeseburgers for dinner. Chain restaurants like Applebee's and Chili's offer numerous burger options that are blessed with bacon. A&W claims to be the first fast-food restaurant to add bacon to a cheeseburger. Sonic Drive-In lets customers add bacon to any sandwich on their menu. McDonald's has served bacon, egg, and cheese sandwiches to billions. When it comes to fast food, your daily bacon dining options are truly unlimited; if a bacon craving suddenly sneaks up on you, chances are you don't need to travel far to satisfy your needs. However, in the last several years, bacon has begun to break out of the fast-food box in a big way.

Bacon owes some of its prominence to the generally heightened interest in food and cooking that has occurred over the last decade. One of the leaders in this movement is the Southern Foodways Alliance, an organization that celebrates American food culture. Given the southern focus, there is not surprisingly a heavy focus on pork products. The SFA Web site even has an entire section dedicated to the history of bacon, and there is also a Web page that lists dozens of recipes for making multiple variations on the BLT sandwich. The SFA hosts several events each year all around the South that people will travel hundreds of miles to attend. Driving hundreds of miles for The Best Meat Ever is a true modern-day pilgrimage.

But these days you don't need to get in your car or board an airplane to experience food culture or to learn more about your beloved bacon. In fact, you don't even need to leave your couch. As the Food Network has increased in popularity, food blogs have become prolific, and celebrity chefs have achieved rock-star status, bacon has also found its way to the top of the food chain.

On the Food Network show *Iron Chef America*, bacon was the secret ingredient of the episode that originally aired on June 4, 2006, pitting Iron Chef Bobby Flay against Toronto chef Susur Lee. During the hour-long duel, the competitors cranked out dishes such as bacon risotto with quail egg and green onion, and Irish bacon–wrapped pork tenderloin—certainly a far cry from traditional food combos like the BLT and spaghetti carbonara that we normally associate bacon with. Comedian Mo Rocca was one of the judges, preventing the competition from becoming too serious or tense. Mo opened up the show by stating that when he was "growing up in my house, we had a quota of four strips of bacon because of health concerns. So this is going to be the most delicious betrayal of my family, to shovel down ten plates of bacon." In judging Chef Flay's deconstructed pancetta carbonara, Rocca quipped that "maybe my imagination is getting away from me, but I just feel like this food is so rich that I'm just gonna die. But it's a great way to go out." This competition ended up in a tie, which makes sense, because when it comes to bacon there are no losers.

A recent addition to the Food Network's Iron Chef lineup is Michael Symon, of the restaurant Lola in Cleveland, Ohio. Chef Symon is also a bacon enthusiast. Oddly enough, he was criticized during the *Iron Chef* audition show that aired on the Food Network in early 2008 (a competition Symon ultimately won) because he made bacon ice cream for the challenge in which contestants were assigned to make desserts with savory ingredients. The problem? That bacon ice cream is nothing new: all of the judges had encountered it before. It was "too safe" and because Symon had made it before, he wasn't being creative enough. That we've reached a point in history at which bacon ice cream is considered to be too conventional speaks volumes about the progress bacon has made in achieving an elevated culinary status in recent years.

Food Network personality Paula Deen, the queen of rich southern fare, is also a big fan of bacon. She's so much of a fan that she is an official spokesperson for Smithfield Foods, one of the largest producers of bacon in the country. On the Smithfield Web site, she once suggested orange-laced french toast casserole with caramelized bacon as a perfect dish to make for Mother's Day. That sounds like a good way to instantly become your mother's favorite child. Paula is also infamous for one of the most sinful dishes you'll ever encounter. Her recipe for a lady's brunch burger consists of a beef patty, fried egg, and two strips of bacon sandwiched between two glazed doughnuts. Your blood pressure might rise just thinking about it, but bless her heart for being so bold in this day and age of culinary political correctness.

Rachael Ray also isn't shy about her love of bacon. The dominatrix of food media regularly features bacon on her television show *30 Minute Meals*, and her magazine, *Every Day Rachael Ray*, is often adorned with bacon-blessed recipes. Like many people, she has her own variations on the BLT sandwich. A recent BLT experiment of hers that was featured in the magazine involved stacking bacon, lettuce, tomato jam, and a thick tuna steak between two slices of bread. Bacon fried rice— a pork belly–inspired variation on a Chinese staple—has also been featured in the magazine. But she doesn't just stick to the bacon basics. She even created her own version of one of Elvis Presley's favorite sandwiches by stuffing bacon, bananas, peanut butter, and honey inside a brioche roll. The heart goes pitter-patter just thinking about it.

While we're on the topic of Elvis's legendary eating habits, the story of his relationship with a sandwich called the Fool's Gold Loaf is one worth sharing. According to legend, Elvis was at home in Memphis one night in February 1976. He was entertaining some guests from

Colorado who began to tell Elvis about a sandwich served by The Colorado Mine Company in Denver that takes overindulgence and launches it into the stratosphere. After having the Fool's Gold sandwich described to him as a single loaf of bread, hollowed out and filled with a jar of peanut butter, a jar of grape jelly, and a pound of bacon, The King decided he needed to experience it immediately. The party drove to the airport, boarded Elvis's private jet, and flew to Denver where they arrived in the middle of the night. They were greeted at the airport by the owners of The Colorado Mine Company, who had brought with them twenty-two loaves for the party to enjoy right there on the spot. Elvis and friends consumed their sandwiches, downed some Champagne, reboarded the plane, and headed back to Memphis before sunrise.

Apparently Elvis isn't the only one who understands the pleasure experienced in combining peanut butter and bacon. There is a strain of everyday citizens who also enjoy this unusual combination. According to a woman named Lisa, a regular reader of Bacon Unwrapped, "a little-known treat to even the most devout bacon disciples is peanut butter and bacon on toast. This is best with several slightly crisp and still warm pieces of bacon so that the peanut butter is converted into smooth, gooey goodness. They are the perfect complement to each other!"

Anthony Bourdain, self-proclaimed archnemesis of Rachael Ray, bane of the Food Network, and—because he embraces such controversy—a popular television personality, is also a big fan of all things pork. Seldom does an episode of his Travel Channel show, *No Reservations*, go by without Tony consuming at least one pork product. And his suggestion to vegetarians? "Try bacon, it's the gateway meat."

Most top chefs will tell you that bacon has always been a staple in their kitchens, even if it wasn't always prominently featured on the menu. But bacon is no longer the redheaded stepchild of high-end kitchens. Bacon is finally getting its turn in the spotlight.

No one embodies the use of bacon in a fine dining establishment better than Grant Achatz, chef and owner of Alinea restaurant in Chicago, and a rising culinary star. His modern approach to dining is demonstrated by his highly creative tasting menu that features an item called Trapeze Bacon. The crispy bacon is garnished with butterscotch, apple, and thyme and then served on a trapeze-like wire that suspends it in midair. Photos of this creation have been circulated throughout the Bacon Nation several times over, making Trapeze Bacon a popular item for food enthusiasts to blog about. Who knew bacon could be as beautiful as it can be delicious.

THE ULTIMATE BACON FANATIC

While there are clearly huge numbers of chefs who love bacon and use it liberally in their cuisine, there is one chef whose obsession lifts him head and shoulders above the rest. That man is Greggory Hill. Formerly of a restaurant called David Greggory in Washington, DC, Chef Hill deserves a lot of credit for bacon's elevated status in restaurants, especially in the nation's capital. His dedication to The Best Meat Ever has helped to put it on the haute cuisine map, not to mention luring unsuspecting innocents into a lifetime membership in the Bacon Nation.

Chef Hill's regular lunch and dinner menus featured several dishes that involved the lovely strips. But what really distinguished him from other bacon-loving chefs were two regular events he hosted at the restaurant. Every Wednesday night he hosted a "Pork and Pinot Happy Hour." But this was no gimmicky restaurant promotion—Chef Hill went out of his way each week to serve a series of small plates, all of which included some form of pork, often in the form of bacon. On those nights, the distinct, tantalizing aroma of bacon wafted out the restaurant's front door—alluring enough to draw in first-time diners, many of whom quickly became loyal patrons.

Chef Hill's ultimate bacon event, however, was his monthly Aphrodisiac Bacon Dinner. This was a 100 percent bacon-focused event with a cult following to match, and was the true embodiment of "bacon as a main event."

The sizzling sound of our favorite meat frying crackled through the air on the night of a bacon dinner. Miniature plastic pigs and other bacon-inspired party favors for the guests decorated the private dining room, and Chef Hill had an impressive display of pig-themed paraphernalia scattered throughout the restaurant to entertain guests waiting to be seated. Also on hand was a representative from The Grateful Palate, a Web site that is a definitive source for artisanal bacons and all of the accoutrements needed to cook and serve that king of meats. The Grateful Palate is the purveyor of the original Bacon of the Month Club (giving your loved ones an annual subscription to the Bacon of the Month Club happens to be a supreme way of expressing affection). The Aphrodisiac Bacon Dinners were the brainchild of Chef Hill and The Grateful Palate's owner, Dan Philips, whose nickname is Captain Bacon.

Besides providing all things bacon, The Grateful Palate also sells Australian wines. So not only did the company provide the bacon and wine for each of Chef Hill's monthly bacon dinners—it sent a representative to serve the guests and describe the wines paired with each course as well. For three hours, diners were served glass upon glass of sumptuous wine to complement course after course of mouth-watering bacon, prepared in a million different ways you could have never imagined yourself. Some of the more memorable bacon dishes served included Grilled Lamb Chops with Petit Jean Bacon-Beet Glaze; Newsom's Smoked Bacon Roulade with Corn Beef, Cabbage, and Vegetable Puree (served at one of the March dinners in honor of St. Patrick's Day); and bacon- and cheese-stuffed pretzel pockets (which are highly, highly addictive).

After Chef Hill's bacon dinners, diners left the restaurant feeling very satisfied, though perhaps a bit like a salt lick (a sensation that, like the wine hangover you also hazarded, had the ability to stick with you into the next day). But the experience was, without a doubt, worth the day of swollen ankles and headaches you might risk.

Chef Hill cast bacon in a sensual light with his Aphrodisiac Bacon Dinners, but he's not the only one who thinks bacon is sexy. Chef Kerry Simon has long had a reputation as a rock 'n' roll chef, and his latest project is CatHouse at the Luxor in Las Vegas. This self-described "world-class restaurant... with an upscale lounge, creating a seductive nightlife venue" is once again reinventing nightlife in Vegas. Part restaurant, part nightclub, CatHouse features several bacon items on its snacking menu. Options for the party set include stuffed mushroom caps with bacon, dates, and blue cheese; an iceberg wedge with applewood smoked bacon; duck confit with roasted beets, goat cheese, candied pecans, dried cherries, and bacon; linguine and mushrooms with radicchio, pancetta, pecans, and Parmesan; and roasted Brussels sprouts with pancetta. Could this possibly be the best nightclub ever to hit Vegas? Can you imagine a better way to spend a night in Vegas than being able to drink a few cocktails, eat some bacon, dance with a few hotties, and then stumble into the casino to play blackjack until the sun rises? It sounds like hedonist heaven.

We could go on and on and on about all of the fabulous restaurants that are doing amazing things with bacon, and all of the wonderful bacon producers who are making their products increasingly available to the general public. But what's really important to recognize here is that bacon is experiencing a culinary renaissance. This is the Golden Age of Bacon. And you don't want to miss it.

CHAPTER 6

BREAKFAST: WHAT BACON KNOWS BEST

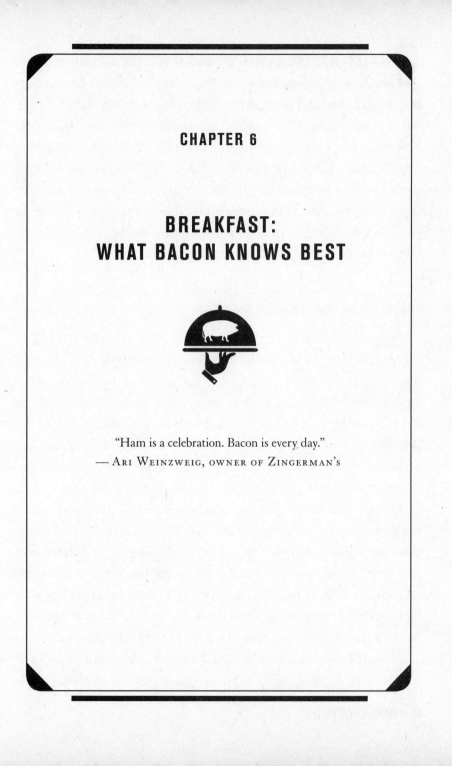

"Ham is a celebration. Bacon is every day."
— ARI WEINZWEIG, OWNER OF ZINGERMAN'S

B REAKFAST IS THE meal at which bacon is the star, where it out-shines eggs, toast, hash browns, sausages, and every other part of the meal that makes breakfast such a delicious experience. When talking about bacon, the conversation almost always revolves around how we like to eat it for breakfast. They may recall fond memories of Sunday morning breakfasts with the family (or the fights over who got the last piece of bacon), frying bacon over a campfire on a cool summer morning in the mountains (but don't do it in bear country—more on that later), or sidling up to the counter at their favorite greasy spoon for breakfast (or at 2:00 A.M. after a night at the bar).

THE KING OF BREAKFAST MEATS

Many people are highly particular about the kind of bacon they like to eat for breakfast. When you're using bacon in another dish, the type doesn't matter as much because the flavor blends in with the other ingredients. But eating a piece on its own is a whole different story. It needs to be the kind of bacon that you think is so delicious it makes you fall in love with the king of breakfast meats over and over again.

When you walk through the meat aisle of any major grocery store in the United States, you will almost always find an entire section dedicated to bacon. And within that section, there are usually several brands to choose from. But it doesn't stop there. Within each of those brands there are options ranging from maple bacon to hickory-smoked bacon to pepper bacon. Then you wander over to the butcher, and they probably have a couple of fresh-cut bacons to consider if you're in the mood for something just a step up from the major brands. When it comes to bacon at the supermarket, there are a multitude of possibilities.

Despite the fact that most people live within a few minutes' drive of such bacon gold mines, there is an increasing trend of consumers seeking out specialty bacons over the Internet, through local butchers, and at farmers' markets. Artisanal bacon is more popular than ever.

Local producers of artisanal bacon have always been around—they predate the major producers most consumers today are familiar with. Newsom's Country Hams, which has been operating a smokehouse in Princeton, Kentucky, since 1917, sells products that have appeared on the menus of some of the top restaurants in the country. Even though they are known best for their hams, their hickory-smoked bacon is equally popular and has its own cult following.

Kentucky—as well as neighboring states Missouri and Tennessee—may have a deep and rich history of local artisans who make bacon, but there are countless butchers around the country who also pride themselves on their cured pork belly. The Pork Shop in Queen Creek, Arizona, is one of the best. The Pork Shop is on the far outskirts of the Phoenix metropolitan area, and for many it is a two-hour round trip from home. But it's the best two hours you could possibly spend in your car, even when it's 115 degrees Fahrenheit outside.

The Pork Shop has been selling top quality pork products to the Valley of the Sun since 1979. The quality and freshness of their pork is why they've been around for so long. They source their hogs locally, with a freshly slaughtered batch arriving on Tuesday and Wednesday each week. And anyone who is familiar with The Pork Shop knows that if you don't show up soon after the meat has been put in the display case, your options will be limited. Bacon, sausages, and chops fly off the shelves at the speed of light at The Pork Shop.

Best of all, the fine folks at The Pork Shop cure their own bacon, which they sell directly to customers at the store. They have a number of bacon products to choose from including hickory-smoked bacon, Kansas City bacon, pepper-cured bacon, Canadian bacon, and bacon ends. A lot of people in Phoenix are familiar with The Pork Shop's bacon without even realizing it and without ever making the pilgrimage to Queen Creek, though. That's because they sell their products to several Phoenix restaurants, including a place called Matt's Big Breakfast—a breakfast joint that is definitely worth getting out of bed and putting on clothes for on a Saturday morning. The Pork Shop's bacon is one of the reasons why breakfast at Matt's is always such a happy experience.

Thielen's Meat Market in Pierz, Minnesota, is another independent butcher that has been providing top-quality meat to residents of central Minnesota since the 1920s. This small town actually had three meat markets at one point—those Minnesotans really do love their bacon! Nowadays, Thielen's is the only meat market still operating in Pierz. Thielen's rose to the top quite simply because of the quality of their product. And recently they've even been recognized for their delicious cured meats by the national media and fanatics all over the country.

As with many butcher shops and smokehouses, Thielen's started out as a custom butcher. But when the business moved to its current location, they quit the butchery business and just started doing processing. Like many independent butchers, Thielen's is a family-owned business run by a father and his sons.

The large custom-built smokehouses in the back of the Thielen's store are quite impressive. When you pull up to the front of the store, you can smell the strong scent of smoking bacon before you even get out of your car.

Thielen's bacon is very popular in this part of the country, and they try to offer their consumers a variety. Andy Thielen, one of the sons—and grandson of the founder of Thielen's Meat Market—explains: "We have regular, double smoked, pepper, and garlic bacon. We tried jalapeño bacon but it just wasn't hot enough. You can do a million different kinds of bacon, but those are the best sellers."

Andy says that like other smokehouses, Thielen's bacon sales have been higher in the last few years. "Our regular bacon is definitely the most popular. I like the garlic myself. But I'm a garlic freak. We cook bacon every morning in the break room for employees to eat. I like to cook it low and slow. Or if you have the patience, outdoor on a wood fire. That's the best."

But you shouldn't have to travel far from home to get your own breakfast bacon from a customer butcher. Some of the best bacons come from small producers who set up shop on weekends at your local farmers' markets. There is a good chance you will be pleasantly surprised by the artisanal bacon options available to you from people who are practically your neighbors.

In New York City at the Union Square Greenmarket, the celebrated Flying Pigs Farm is one of the most popular vendors. Flying Pigs Farm specializes in raising heritage breed pigs—Large Blacks, Gloucestershire Old Spots, and Tamworths. These breeds are becoming increasingly rare in a world dominated by corporate farms, but Flying Pigs owners Michael Yezzi and Jennifer Small are doing their best to preserve them and make their higher quality meat available to more consumers. They also produce nitrate-free bacon in response to demand for such products. Flying Pigs Farm's efforts are gaining recognition—in addition to selling at farmers' markets and over the Internet, their products are in demand at several top restaurants in New York City. They have even received national media attention for their dedication to the art. Pigs will probably never fly, but Flying Pigs Farm bacon will be flying off the shelves for many years to come.

If you don't have a farmers' market in your community, or there aren't any good pork butchers or local artisanal bacon curers near where you live, there are many, many options online for you to choose from. Beyond visiting the individual Web sites of the various niche producers, you can also subscribe to a "Bacon of the Month" club to get a taste of some of the best artisanal bacons currently on the market. These clubs ensure that you are able to have a different delicious bacon-blessed breakfast at least once a month. The purveyors of these monthly clubs get paid to know who has the best bacon so they can offer it to you—tap into their knowledge! The Grateful Palate (Oxnard, California), Zingerman's (Ann Arbor, Michigan), and Coastal Vineyards (Moorpark, California) are a few such clubs that you can learn more about by visiting their Web sites.

FOOD OF THE GODS

The Aztecs were clued into bacon's meaty goodness 800 years ahead of the rest of us. It is said to have been one of the favored dishes of Quetzalcoatl, the Aztec sky and creator god. And if bacon was good enough for him, rest assured that the other denizens of Mesoamerica were chowing down on it, too.

The rock band Foo Fighters are reportedly enamored with pork belly in its cured form. They like to have bacon backstage at every concert, and refer to it as "God's currency." "If it could be breathed, I would," claimed one band member. Bacon in any form is great. Not as an entrée, but just in general."

BACON: A BEAR NECESSITY

While we're on the topic of eating bacon for breakfast, this would be a good time to tell you about the perils of eating bacon for breakfast in bear country. Eric Savage is an entrepreneur who ran a very popular street vendor business for ten years in Boise. Eric owes a lot of his success to bacon, which was served on several of his menu items. But he also has an incredible story that confirms the animal instinct that is our attraction to bacon.

When Eric was a kid, his family had a cabin in eastern Idaho near the border with Yellowstone National Park. The cabin had an indoor grill that vented to the outside. Every morning his father would get up and cook bacon and pancakes for breakfast. One morning, they had just sat down to eat breakfast when suddenly there was a loud noise at the back door of the cabin, right behind where Eric's dad was sitting.

"All of a sudden these big paws came up, grabbed hold of the screen door, and ripped the screen door off the hinges. We could see the bear through the window and it started beating on the door. My dad got his rifle, went out the front door and around to the back of the cabin, and shot the bear. Later we heard that bacon drives bears absolutely nuts. What this bear was doing was so aggressive. The vent going out of the house had sent the bacon smell outside." This kind of reaction to bacon is sometimes also exhibited by the most dedicated members of the Bacon Nation, but even they aren't as scary as a bear on a mission to get its hands on The Best Meat Ever!

Roll forward a few decades to present-day Idaho. Eric does a lot of weeklong backpacking trips in the mountains. "What I used to do for the first night is I'd take a nice steak, wrap it in some bacon, freeze it, and throw it in my backpack. So the first night when I'd get back in there I could cook a nice steak. Where we camp is about fourteen miles in. I'd seen bear markings up there before. But I'd kind of forgotten about the bacon thing that happened with the bear when I was a kid."

"So I was sitting there at nighttime, had just finished cooking up a steak and eating dinner, and it was a pitch-black night—no moon. It was as black as can be. All of a sudden I heard a couple of twigs break behind me, which isn't unusual because there are a bunch of deer in the area. I was there with my girlfriend. So I got my little flashlight and turned around to look, and all I saw were these two red eyes that looked like the devil. It was a bear and he had his nose down, which meant he was hunting. When a bear has its nose down, that's when you have to be the most worried. And he was only about twenty feet from me." And as far as the bear was concerned, it was twenty feet away from a potentially awesome bacon encounter—as scary as this situation was for Eric, what the bear was feeling is something most members of the Bacon Nation can relate to!

"My girlfriend and I jumped up and I grabbed my harmonica and started ripping off a few chords. The bear turned around and ran about twenty feet, and then turned around and started coming back. So I started screaming and hollering. I didn't have a gun with me (I've had one with me every time since). I grabbed the pans off the fire and started banging them together. And the bear ran up to a little ridge that's about fifty feet behind the campsite and ten feet above it. And that bear paced all night long, back and forth. I didn't sleep a wink; it was the scariest night of my life. All that was running through my mind the whole time is that it was the bacon. I hadn't learned that lesson as a kid, and now it was the bacon that brought the bear in. All I had with me was my eight-inch buck knife. Now I carry a .357 and I don't take bacon. Bears and bacon are a very scary combination!"

SOME GUYS WHO ARE DOING IT RIGHT

Swiss Meat and Sausage Company in Hermann, Missouri, makes some of the best bacon that a breakfast lover's money can buy. And the popularity of their cured meats has gained them a lot of national recognition recently. Their big break was a couple of years ago when they were featured on a show on the Food Network. The Food Network had warned them that when the show aired they'd get really busy, but they didn't anticipate the level of response. "The very first time the show aired, we had more than 15,000 requests on our Web site," said owner Mike Sloan. "So we funneled our way through those and got caught up. And then they ran the show again. They ran it ten or twelve times. So we would watch the Internet and when our episode was coming up, we would get ready. And it wasn't our bacon or sausage products we were running out of, it was our dry products—coolers, cardboard boxes, dry ice—things we couldn't make here. But it was a good problem to have!" When the Bacon Nation catches wind of good bacon, there's no holding them back.

Another business that has benefited from the power of the Food Network is Matt's Big Breakfast in Phoenix, Arizona. Not so long ago, Matt's was one of the best-kept secrets in downtown Phoenix. If you didn't live in downtown Phoenix, chances are you had no idea this gem existed. Unfortunately, Matt's is no longer a secret at all. After extensive media coverage and an appearance on the Food Network, the wait to get into the restaurant on a weekend morning can now be more than two hours. And the only place you can wait is outside—including in the middle of summer when it is a scorching hot day in the Sonoran Desert. But devotees will wait because it is just that good. Besides, it's a dry heat (yeah, right . . .).

Matt's Big Breakfast is a family run business. Matt and Erenia Pool are one of the most popular couples in downtown Phoenix thanks to their cheery restaurant, and they're often seen behind the counter serving customers themselves. Their constant presence at the restaurant is particularly impressive because they also own a bar down the street and are often serving wine at 10:00 P.M. to the same customers they served breakfast to at 10:00 A.M. It's a mystery as to when these people sleep because not only do they run two of the most popular businesses in downtown Phoenix but they are personally involved in those businesses on a daily basis. But Phoenicians are grateful for their infinite energy.

Matt's is located in a restored house that is not much more than 1,000 square feet in size—hence the reason for the big lines. The action is centered around an orange 1950s-style bar where the staff ensures that your juice glasses and coffee mugs are always full, regardless of how busy and harried they may be. Even though they'd love to see you eat and run so they can serve more of the customers waiting outside, you never feel rushed. Customers are part of the family at Matt's Big Breakfast.

Matt gets his bacon from the fabulous Pork Shop in Queen Creek, Arizona, which is one very important reason this restaurant is so popular. Their thick-cut bacon is incorporated into a couple of Matt's featured breakfast items. One is the Five Spot, a hearty breakfast sandwich featuring two eggs, two slices of thick-cut bacon, American cheese, and grilled onions on a roll. Another ode to pork is The Hog and Chick—two eggs with a choice of thick-cut bacon, sausage, or off-the-bone ham (tough choice but we all know what the right decision is here). Bacon can also be ordered on the side with any of the other items on the breakfast menu. Despite the restaurant being called Matt's Big Breakfast, they also serve lunch and it is one of the more popular lunch spots for professionals who work downtown Monday through Friday. Not surprisingly, one of the most satisfying items on their lunch menu is the BLT. The BLT at Matt's is made exactly the way BLTs should be made—thick-cut bacon, crispy iceberg lettuce, and juicy vine-ripened tomatoes on thick toasted country bread with real mayonnaise. The juices from the sandwich drip down your arms as you shove it in your mouth. It is a heavenly experience.

For tasty bacon in our nation's capital, try Ben's Chili Bowl, a popular neighborhood establishment since 1958. Ben's is most famous for chili and half-smoke sausages (a native DC delicacy), but their breakfast is equally delicious. There are several bacon options to choose from, including the Bacon and Egg Sandwich or a BLT sandwich. The simplest and most indulgent way to consume bacon for breakfast at Ben's, however, is the Bacon Breakfast. This plate o' heaven comes with two eggs, toast, and an enormous pile of bacon. And "enormous" is no exaggeration—we're talking more than most people can consume in one sitting. It is magnificent.

Simple ingredients and good bacon might be the key to a positive breakfast experience, but that doesn't mean you can't get a little creative. The savory aroma and taste of bacon is a perfect complement to the sweet flavors of pancakes and maple syrup, and the two flavors don't necessarily need to be presented as separate dishes. Bacon pancakes—as in actual bits of bacon cooked into the pancakes—appear on the menus of many breakfast restaurants around the country, most notably The Original Pancake House, a breakfast chain in locations all over the United States. Eating a stack of bacon pancakes topped with whipped butter and drenched in maple syrup is a quick way to put yourself into a food coma and destroy a productive weekend afternoon. So forget going to Home Depot, just eat more bacon pancakes.

However, if you really want to give your cholesterol count a run for its money, try tasting caramelized bacon. There's a good chance you won't be able to stop eating it until you feel like your heart is going to stop. It's just that good. And what's even better is that caramelized bacon is incredibly easy to make at home. Basically all you do is bake some bacon in the oven as you normally would, but beforehand, spread brown sugar all over it. For a little extra kick, sprinkle some chili powder or flakes on top. The result will make you look at bacon in a whole new light. It's like the candied apple version of bacon. Someone needs to figure out a way to put it on a stick and sell it at the state fair. Or on street corners. Just anywhere that we can have easier access. Bring on the caramelized bacon, please!

One restaurant that has perfected the art of caramelized bacon is a bistro called Brick 29 in Nampa, Idaho. Not only do they serve it on the lunch menu in the form of a BLT (you haven't had a good BLT until you've had one made with caramelized bacon) but they also sell it by the trayful at their Sunday brunch, making it both a dangerous and blessed post-church event. Chef Dustan Bristol thinks our love for bacon is a nostalgic thing. "It stems from childhood. The smell of bacon is always a good memory of breakfast, pajamas, and watching cartoons."

Praline bacon (sometimes also called pecan bacon) is another enhanced way to consume your breakfast bacon. This delicacy can sometimes be found at restaurants, particularly in the South. Praline bacon is essentially the same as caramelized bacon except that some chopped pecans also come to the party. Praline bacon is as much a dessert as it is a breakfast item.

As sinfully delicious as caramelized forms of bacon might be, there's one other bacon-blessed breakfast item that makes candied bacon seem pretty tame.

Voodoo Doughnuts in Portland, Oregon, has an entertaining and unconventional approach to making doughnuts. This is not the place to go if you're looking for a simple glazed doughnut. Some of the funkier items on their menu include the Voodoo Doll Doughnut (a doll-shaped doughnut covered in chocolate glaze with a pretzel stick stabbed through where a doughnut's heart might be) and the Dirt (a doughnut covered with vanilla glaze and crumbled Oreo cookies—looks dirty, tastes heavenly). But the item they've become quite famous for recently, thanks largely to a visit by Anthony Bourdain on an episode of the Travel Channel's *No Reservations*, is their bacon maple bar. There's nothing fancy about this pork-themed treat—it is simply a bar-shaped maple doughnut with small strips of bacon on top.

But while the execution may be simple, the concept is brilliant. And Portland doughnut lovers gobble them up almost faster than they can be produced.

According to Kenneth "Cat Daddy" Pogson, owner of Voodoo Doughnuts, the inspiration for the bacon maple (BM) bar evolved out of the desire to make a doughnut that combines savory and sweet flavors, a combination that Cat Daddy feels is very underrated. "The BM became the answer." As you can imagine, the BM has evoked a variety of reactions from customers. One of the best comments, which probably sums up the experience of most people who eat the BM, was "it sounded gross until I took a bite."

The success of the BM has led to other bacon doughnut combo experimentations, including taking a run at the antimeat crowd. "We put Bac-Os Bits on the vegan doughnuts because they contain no meat, but that didn't go over too well. It was just salt and MSG. Some people request bacon on our Memphis Mafia Fritter. That would make it a banana fritter with peanuts, chocolate chips, peanut butter, chocolate frosting, *and* bacon." That definitely sounds like something Elvis and any hard-core member of the Bacon Nation would enjoy.

BACON 365/24/7

Have you ever wondered why breakfast is the only meal people want to have access to all day long? No one ever wants dinner for breakfast. Lunch for dinner would just be lame. But breakfast for lunch or dinner—that's a *real* treat. We want easy access to breakfast so badly that we've even created a meal called brunch just so we can eat breakfast later in the day without feeling like we missed our window of opportunity. And some breakfast joints even offer late-night breakfast hours, which are particularly popular with truck drivers and bar hoppers. Because after a night of partying, the best thing to get you ready for bed (or sober you up before your drive home) is a hearty breakfast.

Bacon isn't just for breakfast, but it is a large reason why the meal is so popular, and it may be why we covet breakfast all day long. It's the only time where you can eat several individual strips of bacon that aren't a part of another dish or sandwich, and no one will judge you. And fortunately there are many establishments that cater to this basic human need.

Denny's is the all-day breakfast joint Americans are most familiar with. For many people, Denny's is an establishment they visit during the morning hours. Other people might not even know what a Denny's looks like before 11:00 p.m. But the beautiful thing about Denny's, no matter what time of day you visit, is that we all have equal access to an All-American Slam (three scrambled eggs with Cheddar cheese, two bacon strips *and* two sausage links, hash browns or grits, and bread) twenty-four hours a day, seven days a week. God Bless America.

Waffle House is also a good spot for those who like to eat bacon for breakfast all day long. All you have to do is pull off practically any interstate exit in the United States and within minutes you can be downing a Grilled Texas Bacon Egg & Cheese Melt.

But Denny's and Waffle House pale in comparison to the gustatory experience that is Cracker Barrel. It's no coincidence that the name Cracker Barrel contains the word "crack" because that's what Cracker Barrel is for many of its regular patrons. When the topic of what to have for breakfast is discussed in middle America, more often than not "Cracker Barrel" flies out of someone's mouth faster than you can say "anywhere with bacon, please." It's a phenomenon not everyone is capable of understanding, much like NASCAR and mullets, but boy, do people like Cracker Barrel. And at Cracker Barrel, you can have their thick-sliced bacon served with a wide variety of other favorite breakfast foods. Any. Time. Of. Day. And *that* is a phenomenon we can all understand and support.

As much as the national chains may appeal to our all-day breakfast and bacon needs, some of the best all-day breakfast joints are locally owned. In Arlington, Virginia, Bob & Edith's is a classic diner that has been serving the 24/7 breakfast crowd for many years. The diner is very small, yet people will wait in line to get a seat, even at 2:00 A.M. Because if you've been out having a good time with your friends and you need a hit of tasty bacon before you go home, you'll wait for that hit—no matter what time of day it is, rain or shine. Breakfast is the best meal ever, bacon is The Best Meat Ever, and they are both appropriate anytime, anywhere, at (almost) any cost.

GETTING DOWN TO THE BUSINESS OF MAKING BREAKFAST

So now you know all about where to get the best breakfast with The Best Meat Ever if you happen to be on the road. But what about when you're staying at home and hankering for homemade breakfast with a jolt of bacon magnificence? What should you make and, quite frankly, why should you go to the trouble? The possibilities are limited only by your own imagination, and the mere thought of putting a bacon-blessed breakfast together should serve as enough inspiration for you to concoct a meal that will get your day off to the right start. One of the many things that makes this ritual so enjoyable (and you know it!) is the smell of frying bacon. When you sink your teeth into your first slice of bacon, the day can officially begin.

There are countless ways of preparing bacon for breakfast. A standard breakfast of bacon with eggs on the side is always nice, but it's also fun to combine all of your breakfast ingredients into pizzas, burritos, and sandwiches. And these combinations could not be any easier to make.

Breakfast pizzas can be made either as an individual serving or as one large pizza for a group to share. If you don't have the time or energy to make your own dough, stop by your local grocery store the night before to pick up a premade selection. There are many frozen brands available, but if you can find a store that sells it fresh, all the better.

You can assemble the breakfast pizza with any of your favorite breakfast toppings—the options are almost limitless since bacon goes with pretty much any ingredient you would eat for breakfast. Be creative and try a combination of salty and sweet flavors—apples with bacon is a good one. Or, if you're in a traditional mood, stick with a combination of basic ingredients. To make a simple breakfast pizza, flatten the dough, brush it with oil, and place it on a baking sheet. Then layer the dough with toppings you've cooked ahead of time such as scrambled eggs and crumbled bacon. Next add shredded Colby Jack cheese on top. That's it—it's simple, quick, and doesn't require a lot of brainpower early in the morning. Bake the pizza at 450°F for 8 to 10 minutes. You'll be able to scarf it down in less time than it took you to make the pizza, and then you can start the day.

Breakfast burritos are another delicious breakfast no-brainer. Once again—you can use any ingredients you like. But one of the best ways to make a breakfast burrito is to keep it simple, just like a breakfast pizza. To assemble a basic breakfast burrito, start by scrambling some eggs. Then fry and crumble some bacon, place the eggs and bacon on a tortilla, top it with cheese, wrap it up, and throw it into the microwave for 30 seconds to warm up the tortilla and melt the cheese. You can garnish the burrito with ingredients such as sour cream, black olives, and salsa. From the time the ingredients come out of the refrigerator until they are in your belly is usually less than ten minutes. And that is by far the best part of the meal (after the bacon, of course).

Keeping with the simple theme, this author's favorite breakfast sandwich is also a breeze to make. The sandwich was discovered while on vacation on the Hawaiian island of Maui several years ago. At a roadside café on the beach near Hana, they served a breakfast sandwich that is so simple it is absolutely brilliant. The sandwich is merely an arrangement of scrambled eggs, American cheese, and two strips of bacon on a sesame-seed hamburger bun. The fact that it was enjoyed on a beautiful beach looking out at the Pacific Ocean made it a truly magical experience.

So breakfast can be delicious without being complicated. That is the beauty of breakfast. And it is one reason why bacon is such an integral part of the meal—it's a simple, uncomplicated meat that is just plain tasty. Here are a few more recipes to get your early morning motor running.

EGG CASSEROLE

Egg Casserole plays a very important role at Lauer family gatherings. The author's mother has been preparing it for Christmas breakfast for decades, and even though the author is not a morning person, the smell of frying bacon and Egg Casserole baking in the oven are the only two things that get her out of bed on Christmas morning. Egg Casserole really doesn't need anything to make it better, but bacon does add a whole new level of enjoyment to the experience, if that's even possible. Egg Casserole is seriously that delicious, so be prepared to slip into a food coma after your third serving and sleep your way through to dinner. Wear pants with an elastic waistband. You've been warned.

4 tablespoons (½ stick) salted butter, melted, plus extra for
   the baking dish
6 slices sourdough bread, crust removed and cubed
½ pound Velveeta cheese, cubed
3 large eggs, beaten
2 cups milk
½ teaspoon dry mustard
Pinch of salt
Pinch of pepper
10 slices bacon, cut into ½-inch pieces

1. Butter an 8-inch square baking dish. Layer the bread and cheese
   in the baking dish. In a medium bowl, whisk together the eggs,
   milk, melted butter, dry mustard, salt, and pepper. Pour the
   mixture over the bread and cheese. Cover with plastic wrap and
   refrigerate overnight.
2. The next morning, preheat the oven to 350°F. Sprinkle the
   bacon over the top. Bake uncovered for 1 hour. Serve while hot
   and gooey.

BACON BISCUITS

This recipe is from Chef Greggory Hill, formerly of the restaurant David Greggory in Washington, DC. These biscuits can be eaten just as they are, or per Chef Hill's recommendation, sliced open and filled with a couple of strips of bacon.

MAKES 8 TO 10 BISCUITS

¼ pound bacon, cut into ½-inch pieces
2 cups all-purpose flour, plus extra for the work surface
½ teaspoon sugar
1 teaspoon kosher salt
½ teaspoon baking powder
¼ teaspoon baking soda
1 teaspoon active dry yeast
1 teaspoon ground black pepper
8 tablespoons (1 stick) butter, cut into small dice and chilled
¼ cup cold water
1 cup buttermilk
Nonstick cooking spray

1. Place a cast-iron or other heavy skillet over medium heat. Cook the bacon slowly, stirring occasionally to prevent sticking. Once the fat is rendered and the bacon is crispy, remove the bacon with a slotted spoon to a paper towel–lined plate. Transfer the drippings to a container and reserve.

2. Sift the flour, sugar, salt, baking powder, and baking soda into a large bowl. Stir in the yeast and black pepper. With a fork, blend in the butter and 6 tablespoons of the drippings until the mixture looks like coarse meal. Stir in the cold water and buttermilk just until mixed. Fold in the bacon. Cover the bowl with a kitchen

towel or plastic wrap and allow to rise at room temperature for 45 minutes to 1 hour.

3. Preheat the oven to 350°F. Lightly spray a baking sheet with cooking spray.

4. Turn the dough out of the bowl onto a lightly floured work surface. Dust the dough with a little more flour and use a rolling pin to flatten it to 1/4 inch thick. Cut out biscuits with a 1- to 2-inch biscuit cutter or a small glass and place the cut biscuits on the baking sheet (it's OK if the biscuits touch). Reroll the dough scraps and repeat until all the dough has been cut. Bake for 10 to 12 minutes, until golden on the top and sides. Serve hot from the oven, with or without extra bacon (with is better).

BACON FRITTATA

Rocco Loosbrock of Coastal Vineyards and his recipe guru, Brenda Beaman, developed this recipe for a yummy bacon frittata that is a great dish for breakfast, lunch, or dinner—or any time in between. This can be served hot, at room temperature, or cold.

SERVES 8

½ pound bacon, cut into ½-inch pieces
8 ounces fresh mushrooms, trimmed, wiped clean, and sliced
Nonstick cooking spray
10 large eggs, lightly beaten, or 2 cups egg substitute
1 cup shredded smoked Gouda cheese (¼ pound)
2 medium tomatoes, seeded and chopped
1 green onion (scallion), trimmed and chopped

1. Preheat the oven to 350°F.

2. Cook the bacon in a large heavy skillet over medium-high heat, stirring constantly, until the fat has rendered and the bacon is cooked to your preferred doneness. Remove the bacon with a slotted spoon to a paper towel–lined plate.

3. Add the mushrooms to the fat in the skillet. Cook the mushrooms, stirring occasionally, until they have stopped giving up water and are uniformly golden brown. Set aside.

4. Liberally spray a 10-inch ovenproof skillet with nonstick cooking spray. Heat the skillet over medium-high heat. Pour in about one third of the eggs and let cook briefly to set the bottom. Evenly sprinkle on the bacon, mushrooms, and cheese. Pour in the remaining eggs. Cook the frittata without stirring just until small bubbles come to the top. Transfer to the oven and bake until the eggs are completely set, 10 to 15 minutes.

5. Remove the frittata from the oven and allow it to rest for at least 5 minutes. Cut it into 8 pieces and serve topped with fresh tomatoes and a sprinkle of green onion.

HANA BEACH BREAKFAST SANDWICH

This particular variation on a bacon, egg, and cheese breakfast sandwich was inspired by a sandwich found at a roadside café near the beach town of Hana on the Hawaiian island of Maui. It's simple, it's hearty, it's delicious.

SERVES 1

2 slices bacon (your favorite brand and variety)
1 sesame-seed hamburger bun, split
2 eggs
Butter (optional)
2 slices American (or your favorite) cheese

Cook the bacon by your preferred method to your desired level of crispiness; set aside on a paper towel–lined plate. Toast the hamburger bun in a small skillet in the bacon drippings or plain in a toaster oven. Set aside to keep warm. Scramble the eggs to your preferred texture in the skillet in the bacon drippings or in butter, if using. Pile the eggs, bacon, and cheese on one side of the bun, place the other side of the bun on top, lift the sandwich to your mouth, and savor every last bite.

CHAPTER 7

WRAPPED IN BACON

"Bacon isn't a food, it's a flavor."
—John Martin Taylor, food historian, writer,
and owner of Hoppin' John's culinary Web site

DO YOU EVER wonder who the first person was to wrap something in bacon? Whoever this person was, they were clearly a genius and well ahead of their time. And they must have had a serious bacon obsession, because why else would someone come up with the idea to make another food better by wrapping it with bacon? The only sensible conclusion is that this individual believed that bacon had the power to make everything it enveloped that much more delicious. Whatever the motivation, the result was utterly brilliant and the concept has since been enthusiastically accepted and executed in hundreds of splendid ways.

MEAT-WRAPPED MEAT

Chef Greggory Hill of Washington, DC, has his own take on the allure of wrapping other foods in bacon:

> *It adds so much flavor to any dish. Take shrimp, which is kind of bland in flavor, and wrap a piece of smoky bacon around it and watch it take on a whole different characteristic. Same with scallops or anything else you wrap with it . . . bacon wakes things up and gives the food a whole smoky characteristic. The flavors come to life.*

The cocktail party where bacon-wrapped shrimp first made an appearance must have been the best cocktail party ever. Those partygoers probably showed up hoping that an open bar would help get them through an evening full of meaningless chitchat and then *shazam!*—out come the bacon-wrapped shrimp. The hosts probably couldn't fill the trays fast enough. Just imagine hands grabbing and elbows jabbing and bacon-wrapped shrimp being shoved into mouths by the handful with the leftover tails littering the carpet. Suddenly it's 2:00 A.M., everyone has bacon grease smeared all over their suits and cocktail dresses, and the hosts have to start kicking people out and calling taxis. That was, clearly, a cocktail party for the ages.

The best bacon-wrapped shrimp this author has ever encountered weren't at a cocktail party at all, but rather at a restaurant called Richardson's in Phoenix, Arizona. A few things set these bacon-wrapped shrimp apart from the rest. Six jumbo shrimp are wrapped in Nueske's bacon and grilled over an open fire. The result is a crispy piece of bacon wrapped around a juicy shrimp with slightly burnt edges. But it gets even better. The grilled shrimp are then served on a warm plate with a fresh tortilla, rice, pinto beans, and three dipping sauces—jalapeño hollandaise, red chili, and salsa. The flavor combinations explode in your mouth—it is a full-on religious experience. You experience spicy, sweet, savory, and salty all at once (have you ever noticed that many of the words used to describe the flavors of food start with an *S*?). The bacon-wrapped shrimp at Richardson's is one of the best culinary experiences in the southwestern United States. You'll laugh, you'll cry, you'll waddle to your car happy. You might even want to consider finding a designated driver just in case you pass out from a happy food coma on the ride home.

Shrimp isn't the only food that benefits from a relationship with bacon. Steak is another suitable companion for The Best Meat Ever. Imagine the first restaurant to serve a bacon-wrapped filet mignon. You can just envision some steak snob's mind being blown when they discover that a strip of cured pork belly is strangling their precious prime cut, yet they can't put their fork down because it's the most delicious thing they've ever encountered, and it makes them feel a little bit naughty and perhaps they're even a bit turned on. Humans have increasingly caught on to the pleasure of combining steak and bacon over the years, and now you can hardly step foot in a chain restaurant or upscale steakhouse without encountering bacon-wrapped filet mignon on the menu. And bacon-wrapped steak is one of the easiest and most delightful things to throw on the grill at home. It is perfect for summertime cookouts and is a guaranteed crowd pleaser (just don't take it camping with you in bear country).

Chicken is no different. On its own, a chicken breast can be all delicious and healthy and stuff. But wrap a piece of bacon around it and the saltiness of the bacon makes the chicken a thousand times more enjoyable. Not only does bacon make chicken taste better but it also helps it to cook better by helping to keep some of the juices inside the chicken breast that might otherwise be lost during the cooking process. Talk about a multitalented meat. There's really nothing better than a juicy chicken breast seductively enveloped by a gorgeous strip of bacon.

THE BACON DOG

While we're on the topic of bacon-wrapped meats, let's spend a moment talking about bacon-wrapped hot dogs and sausages. This concept is relatively foreign to many Americans, but the practice of wrapping encased meat with bacon has been around for quite some time. In German-speaking countries, this delicacy is often referred to as *Berner Würstel*. Reportedly invented in Austria in the 1950s, the Berner Würstel is a cheese-stuffed sausage wrapped in bacon and fried. It's so delicious that you'll want to yodel from the top of the nearest mountain after tasting one for the first time. And then immediately call your cardiologist.

North America has its own version of bacon-wrapped encased meat. Bacon-wrapped hot dogs might not be familiar to all Americans, but people who live in Arizona and California know this popular street food well. "Bacon dogs" are apparently one of the numerous culinary delights for which we have Mexico to thank. If you've ever traveled around the Mexican states of Baja California or Sonora, there's a good chance you've encountered a bacon dog stand. In Los Angeles, these salty delights are most commonly sold by street vendors. Bacon dogs are exactly what they sound like—a hot dog wrapped in bacon, served on a bun.

While much less common, it's possible to find bacon dogs outside of the Southwest. Crif Dogs, a restaurant in New York City, is famous (or infamous, depending on your personal taste) for their creative bacon-wrapped hot dogs. Their menu features items such as the Chihuahua, a bacon-wrapped hot dog covered with avocados and sour cream (it's way better than you might initially think). For fans of Korean food, there is the Chang, a bacon-wrapped hot dog topped with kimchee (for those who are obsessed with this Korean delicacy, the Chang is a culinary dream team). The Chang's namesake is David Chang, chef of the restaurant Momofuku Ssäm Bar, also located in New York City, and supplier of the kimchee for this creation. And then there's the Crif Dog's version of the bacon dog called the BLT—a bacon-wrapped dog topped with lettuce, tomatoes, and mayo. You have absolutely no idea how amazing this combination is until you've tried it. Mayonnaise, tomatoes, bacon, and hot dogs—who knew it could be so good?

Bacon dogs have gained some national media attention recently because the act of selling bacon-wrapped hot dogs on the streets of Los Angeles has become just about as illegal as selling heroin. Yes, you read that correctly—street vendors can sell hot dogs, they just can't be wrapped in bacon. Apparently some "public health expert" (read: overpaid bureaucrat) within the bowels of the all-knowing Los Angeles County Health Department decided one day that street vendor carts are good enough to store and cook hot dogs, but they aren't good enough to store and cook bacon. Eh??? And because of these so-called bacon-unfriendly carts, street vendors aren't allowed to serve bacon dogs unless they spend thousands of dollars to buy a new state-of-the-art cart. Sounds like the manufacturers of these new carts have some good lobbyists.

What has happened, which is what often happens when the government tries to play nanny, is that licensed street vendors are fined and/or arrested if they are caught selling bacon on their hot dogs. But unlicensed street vendors are popping up all over the place to capitalize on the continued demand for bacon dogs. The unlicensed vendors can disappear as quickly as they appear, and they change locations daily to prevent being caught. The unknowing customer might not have any idea whether a vendor is licensed or not. And even if they did know, chances are they aren't going to let anything get in the way of their bacon dog, including a pesky license. So in an effort to make street food safer for Angelinos, the city government is actually making food less safe. And bacon is unfairly caught in the middle.

If you live in Los Angeles and want to find a safe, street-legal bacon dog, Pink's Hot Dogs is the place to go. Pink's is an L.A. institution, established in 1939 as a hot dog stand on the corner of La Brea and Melrose, and now located in a small building at the same spot. The popularity of Pink's has grown exponentially over the years—far more than the space can handle at times. Outrageous lines are not uncommon. Originally famous for chili dogs, Pink's offers a Bacon Chili Cheese Dog variation on the classic. But that's not your only bacon dog option. The Mulholland Drive Dog—named after the infamous hillside road in L.A.—is a ten-inch-long hot dog with grilled onions, mushrooms, nacho cheese, and bacon. There's also the Bacon Burrito Dog—a flour tortilla wrapped around two hot dogs with cheese, three slices of bacon, chili, and onions. You can upgrade your Bacon Burrito

Dog to a Poli Bacon Burrito Dog by adding a Polish dog to the mix. Pink's has also expanded their menu to offer hamburgers, including the Poli-Bacon Chili Cheeseburger—a grilled Polish dog on a hamburger bun with bacon. In your face, L.A. Health Department.

THE BACON BLOGOSPHERE

In addition to Bacon Unwrapped, several other bloggers dedicate their daily musings to The Best Meat Ever.

- **I ❤ Bacon** (www.iheartbacon.com) was the original bacon blog. It's no longer actively updated, but the legacy lives on.

- **Since 2005, The Bacon Show** (baconshow.blogspot.com) has promised to share "one bacon recipe per day, every day, forever," providing an important service to bacon lovers worldwide.

- **The Bacon Salt Blog** (baconsaltblog.com) offers numerous suggestions for ways to enhance the flavor of anything you eat with their bacon-flavored salts. The inventors of this product also recently released a bacon-flavored mayonnaise called Baconnaise. It makes you wonder where their devotion to creating bacon-flavored condiments will go next.

- **Mr. Baconpants** (WWW.MRBACONPANTS.COM) does indeed own a pair of pants that look like strips of bacon. And this enthusiast doesn't just hide behind the wall of his blog—he's not afraid to don his bacon pants in public at baconcentric events.

- **Skulls and Bacon** (skullsandbacon.blogspot.com) combines the unusual hobbies of eating bacon and collecting skull-themed paraphernalia. Once again proving that everything is better with bacon, even skulls.

THE RIGHT CUT

The key to wrapping something in bacon starts with figuring out the right cut of bacon. There are a variety of cuts available, but the one most consumers are familiar with is the commercial presliced kind found in packages in the meat aisle of your local grocery store. There's also the locally cured presliced bacon in the butcher section of most stores, often a step up from the prepackaged version. For purposes of wrapping most foods in bacon, these prepackaged or butcher options are sufficient.

However, if you need a thinner cut of bacon for wrapping something in particular, such as shrimp or something that is smaller in size, you might want to find a local butcher that sells bacon by the slab so you can get it sliced to order or take it home and slice it yourself (recommended only if you're a serious home cook lucky enough to own a meat slicer).

The concept of wrapping everything and anything in bacon is more popular than ever. Many restaurants with seafood on their menu have evolved well beyond the traditional option of bacon-wrapped shrimp; now you can find many types of fish wrapped in bacon, most often trout, halibut, and salmon. If bacon isn't enough pig for you to consume in one sitting, bacon-wrapped pork loin provides double the pork pleasure. Perhaps you aren't a fan of vegetables, but you know you need to include them in your diet? If so, bacon-wrapped asparagus or bacon-wrapped corn on the cob taste great when prepared on an outdoor grill. Bacon-wrapped figs are now regularly appearing on restaurants' appetizer menus around the country, as are bacon-wrapped water chestnuts. "Water chestnuts?" you ask. If you're feeling skeptical, don't. Until you've dipped this perfectly crispy, salty, crunchy, and strangely refreshing hors d'oeuvre into a bowl of honey, you just haven't lived.

A BACON-WRAPPED BACON FESTIVAL

There's nothing too shocking about wrapping seafood, vegetables, or other meats in bacon. Most anyone who enjoys bacon has encountered those variations on at least one occasion. But there is a movement afoot to find new and unusual ways to wrap other favorite foods. One such example hails from the High Life Lounge in Des Moines, Iowa, a bar that serves a bacon-wrapped Tater Tot appetizer that has developed a cult-like following. This dish consists of the Tot, bacon, a jalapeño pepper, and cheese.

"The jalapeños really put them over the top. They are one of our most popular appetizers and have been featured in a few articles in Des Moines newspapers," said Jeff Bruning, one of the proprietors of the High Life Lounge.

The best thing about bacon-wrapped Tater Tots is that they could not be any easier to make. And one of the best kinds of bacon to use is wild boar bacon from D'Artagnan, a supplier of fine foods. The worst thing about wild boar bacon is that it comes pretty close to ruining all other bacons for anyone who tries it—this stuff is amazing, and it's unfortunate that it isn't more widely available. Wild boar bacon has all of the attributes that make bacon so popular—salty and sweet flavors absorbed by a perfect balance of meat and fat. It also has a certain gaminess to it that appeals to some deep primal instinct. Besides the taste, what makes this D'Artagnan wild boar bacon perfect for bacon-wrapped Tater Tots is that it comes in shorter, thinner strips, just the perfect size for wrapping around a Tater Tot. It's almost as if the wild boar bacon were made just for this purpose.

The entry on Bacon Unwrapped about wild boar bacon–wrapped Tater Tots has continued to be the most popular item on the blog since the day it was published. Dozens of Web sites have linked to the entry, tens of thousands of people have read it, and it has captured the hearts and minds of countless bacon enthusiasts. Perhaps the interest comes from the sinful, subversive nature of combining two foods that are considered by so many people to be politically incorrect. Or maybe it's because everyone loves bacon, and everyone loves Tater Tots, and it only makes sense to bring the two together to create one of the most delicious things you could ever serve at a Super Bowl party. All you need to know is that bacon-wrapped Tater Tots are awesomely delicious.

The popularity of the High Life Lounge bacon-wrapped Tater Tots made it the perfect venue for a festival dedicated to The Best Meat Ever. The event, dubbed the Blue Ribbon Bacon Festival, is the brainchild of local resident Brooks Reynolds.

Back in 2007, Brooks shared his idea for a bacon festival with Jeff Bruning, who simply replied, "We can make that happen." A committee called the Iowa Lard Council was formed, the event was planned, tickets went on sale (and quickly sold out), and 750 pounds of bacon were shipped to the High Life Lounge.

The first-ever Blue Ribbon Bacon Festival was a huge success. Naturally, bacon-wrapped Tater Tots were served throughout the day. But Brooks and Jeff agree about the real highlight. "The bacon eating contest was hilarious (and can be found on YouTube)," says Brooks. Why was the event so popular? Besides the fact that we're talking about The Best Meat Ever, it also helps that Iowans are proud of their hog heritage. "Since there are almost 17 million pigs in the state, we eat a lot of pork," explains Jeff. "Iowans love bacon and when they were told about the bacon fest they were so excited they couldn't wait for the event to happen. We sold the event out before we opened up ticket sales."

With bacon-wrapped Tater Tots, we can see that when it comes to bacon combinations, there's no reason to hold back. Maybe you've thought about wrapping cheese curds with bacon but were afraid to try for fear of creating a mess in your microwave. Fear not—even if you make a mess, it's worth the cleanup that might be involved. Perhaps bacon-wrapped meat loaf is a comfort food you dream about at night. Bacon-wrapped baked apples? It may sound crazy, but these two flavors are very good together. Use your imagination. Go hog wild. Have some fun wrapping the world in bacon.

BACON-WRAPPED TATER TOTS

D'Artagnan Wild Boar Bacon works great for this recipe, but since it is available only through specialty stores or the D'Artagnan Web site, you can replace it with regular bacon here. If you do get your hands on some wild boar bacon, use one slice for each Tater Tot (rather than the half-slice of standard length bacon).

SERVES 2 TO 3

10 slices bacon (your choice), cut in half
20 Ore-Ida Tater Tots
Ketchup and mayonnaise
Dill pickles (optional)

1. Preheat the oven to 425°F. Wrap a half-slice of bacon around each Tater Tot. Place the Tots on a rimmed baking sheet (to catch the bacon grease so it does not drip off the sheet in the oven). Bake for 15 to 18 minutes, until the Tots are golden and crispy and the bacon is cooked. Remove from the oven and put the Tots on a paper towel–lined plate to drain the excess bacon grease.

2. Mix equal parts of ketchup and mayonnaise to create a "special dipping sauce" for your Tots. And call me crazy, but I also like to

serve my bacon-wrapped Tots with dill pickles. As soon as the Tots are cool to the touch (but they taste best warm so make sure they don't cool too much), dip them in the special sauce and enjoy!

SMOKY BACON-WRAPPED DENVER OMELET

The only thing better than an omelet is an omelet wrapped in bacon. Brenda Beaman, "The Pancake Lady," came up with this idea for a hearty bacon-encased breakfast.

SERVES 4

16 to 20 slices bacon (your favorite)
4 large eggs
¼ cup minced red bell pepper
¼ cup minced green bell pepper
¼ cup minced white onion
½ cup grated Cheddar cheese (2 ounces)

1. Preheat the oven to 350°F. Cook the bacon in a skillet on low to medium heat (or in the oven at 350°F for 15 to 20 minutes for faster results) until it is fully cooked but still flexible and not browned. Drain on a paper towel–lined plate. Line four 4-ounce ramekins with 4 to 5 slices of bacon each so that the cups are completely lined with bacon. Create a radial pattern, like spokes of a wheel, with the bacon overlapped in the center and the ends sticking up over the edges of the cup.

2. Beat the eggs until frothy and pour an equal amount into each bacon-lined ramekin. Mix the red bell pepper, green bell pepper, and onion together in a small bowl. Add 2 tablespoons of the vegetable mixture to the eggs in each ramekin. Set aside the remain-

ing vegetable mixture. Gently fold the bacon down over the top of the eggs. Bake the omelets in the oven for about 18 minutes, until the eggs are slightly puffed.

3. Allow the baked omelets to rest for about 5 minutes. Remove them from the ramekins with a spoon and transfer them to serving plates. Garnish each omelet with 2 tablespoons cheese and 1 tablespoon of the reserved vegetable mixture.

INSIDE-OUT CHICKEN CORDON BLEU WITH DIJON DIPPING SAUCE

Stuff some bacon and cheese inside a chicken breast and it's a classic French dish. Wrap the bacon around the outside of the chicken instead, and it becomes a bacon-encased renegade delight. Recipe courtesy of Brenda Beaman.

SERVES 4 AS AN APPETIZER

8 strips bacon
4 frozen breaded chicken tenders, thawed
2 slices deli-cut Swiss cheese

FOR THE DIJON DIPPING SAUCE

2 tablespoons light mayonnaise
2 tablespoons light sour cream
2 teaspoons Dijon mustard
¼ teaspoon grated garlic
1½ teaspoons cream sherry
Freshly ground black pepper

1. Preheat the oven to 350°F. Line a rimmed baking sheet with aluminum foil.

2. Cook the bacon in a large skillet on low to medium heat until it is fully cooked but still flexible and not browned. Set aside to drain on a paper towel–lined plate.

3. Cut the chicken tenders in half lengthwise. Wrap one strip of bacon around each chicken portion in a corkscrew fashion. Place each bacon-wrapped chicken piece on the prepared baking sheet, tucking the ends of the bacon under the chicken. Bake for 15 to 20 minutes, until the chicken is cooked through to the center.

4. While the chicken is cooking, prepare the Dijon dipping sauce by stirring together the mayonnaise, sour cream, mustard, garlic, and sherry in a small serving bowl. Sprinkle the sauce with black pepper.

5. Cut each slice of cheese into 4 strips and set aside. When the chicken is cooked, remove it from the oven and place one strip of cheese on top of each chicken portion. Place the chicken back into the oven for 1 to 2 minutes, until the cheese has begun to melt. Arrange the chicken pieces on a plate with the Dijon dipping sauce and serve.

BACON-WRAPPED WATER CHESTNUTS
DIPPED IN HONEY

When asked, most people probably couldn't tell you where a water chestnut comes from. But it doesn't matter, because when wrapped in a strip of bacon, this starchy vegetable becomes a delicious vehicle for The Best Meat Ever. Dip the bacon-wrapped water chestnuts in some honey to experience sweet and salty pleasure.

SERVES 2 TO 3

20 whole water chestnuts (peeled fresh or drained canned)
10 strips bacon, cut in half crosswise
Honey

Preheat the oven to 350°F. Line a rimmed baking sheet with aluminum foil. Wrap each water chestnut with a half-strip of bacon and secure the bacon with a toothpick. Place on the baking sheet. Bake for 15 to 20 minutes until the bacon is cooked. Drain briefly on a paper towel–lined plate. Dip the water chestnuts in your favorite honey and enjoy.

BACON-WRAPPED CORN ON THE COB

This summertime favorite combines a nutritious serving of corn with your favorite bacon. Recipe courtesy of Rocco Loosbrock of Coastal Vineyards.

SERVES 4

Chili powder
4 ears corn, shucked, silk removed
8 slices hickory-smoked bacon (or your favorite bacon)

Preheat a barbecue grill. Evenly sprinkle chili powder over a square sheet of aluminum foil. Roll an ear of corn in the chili powder to coat it. Wrap two pieces of bacon around the corn. Wrap the corn in the foil and crimp each end. Repeat with the other 3 ears of corn. Place the foil-wrapped corn on the barbecue for about 20 minutes, rolling once or twice. Unwrap the corn and enjoy!

CHAPTER 8

ENHANCED BY BACON

"Bits of bacon are like the fairy dust of the food community. You don't want this baked potato? Brrring! Now it's your favorite part of the meal. Not interested in the salad? Bibbity bobbity BACON. I just turned it into an entrée."
—COMEDIAN JIM GAFFIGAN

WRAPPING SOMETHING ISN'T the only way to enhance the flavor of a particular food or dish with bacon. There are countless other ways to use bacon as a flavor enhancer, ranging from bacon bits on your salad to bacon on your hamburger to cubes of bacon thrown into a pasta sauce that is also held together with bacon grease. You can even carry a bottle of Bacon Salt around in your purse or backpack so that you always have the flavor of bacon at your fingertips. Bacon is the ultimate flavor enhancer, and there are many ways to go about getting your fix.

THE "CHICK BACON ON A TATER"

Someone who is very familiar with the power that bacon has over humans is Eric Savage. Most people would have no reason to know who Eric is. But if you've ever been to the bars in downtown Boise, Idaho, then chances are pretty good you know him well, and at some point you might have even told him you love him. We'll come back to that in a moment.

Idaho is one of those states that most people have never been to. As a result, there are a lot of well-kept secrets when it comes to all of the wonderful sights and experiences Idaho has to offer, including the downtown street vendor scene at night. In the span of just a few blocks of downtown Boise there are several bars that are quite popular on weekends. Given the proximity of these bars to each other, all bar goers end up on the same sidewalk in front of the bars at some point during the evening. And on that sidewalk exists a street vendor community that satisfies the 2:00 A.M. food cravings of the spirited masses.

But the members of this community aren't just your average street vendors. Most of them actually serve really good products, ranging from tacos to hot dogs to chorizos (Idaho has a large population of people whose families originated from the Basque regions of Spain and France, and chorizos are as common in Boise as hot dogs). For ten years, Eric Savage was one of the most popular street vendors on the block.

Eric is a very entrepreneurial fellow who has owned several successful businesses over the course of his career. Before retiring to Arizona in 2006, he spent a decade on the streets of Boise selling a product called the Chick Bacon on a Tater. And the bar crowd *loved* this Idaho-inspired delicacy.

The Chick Bacon on a Tater isn't a complicated concept—that's really the beauty of it. Eric takes a potato that has been infused with a barbecue flavor and wraps it in a tortilla with a piece of chicken breast, a few strips of bacon, and melted cheese. Basically it's the perfect drunk food. He initially came up with the idea one day when he was using his secret infusion method to barbecue potatoes for some friends and family at home. Everyone raved about his potatoes, so he started to think about a strategy for starting a company that capitalized on his ability to infuse potatoes with different flavors.

One day Eric was sitting around wondering how to package his delicious barbecued potatoes and he noticed some hot dog buns in the cupboard. So he started to wonder what the potatoes might taste like on a hot dog bun. He put one of the potatoes on a bun, put some condiments on it, and decided to have a few people over to taste his invention. Everyone thought they were brilliant. So he started working on a recipe to mass-produce his flavored potatoes and began to build hot dog carts from which he could sell his masterpieces.

Eric started out with tater dogs, tater tacos, and, later, hot dogs and chorizos. But he didn't just stop there. "I'm a big bacon fan. We always have bacon at our house. I'll cook up four or five pounds of bacon on my George Foreman grill and put it in bags in the refrigerator. We have bacon like we have butter. But no one was selling bacon on the street. None of the food you sell on the sidewalk can be raw—everything has to be precooked. Around the time I started thinking about this, the stores started coming out with precooked bacon and precooked chicken breasts." A light went on in Eric's head. And the Chick Bacon on a Tater was born.

"I thought, 'What if I did a tater, a chicken breast, and some bacon inside a tortilla?' I did that and it was unbelievable. And I also started putting bacon on my regular hot dogs. When I added the bacon to my business, it increased revenues 35 to 40 percent. Because not only did I have the smell of the barbecue sauce but I also had the smell of bacon. So between the two, people were, well . . . bacon is almost like an aphrodisiac. People just go crazy from the smell of bacon." Yes, Eric, yes they do.

During his ten years on the streets of Boise, Eric enjoyed a wildly successful business at which he only had to work three nights per week in order to make a very comfortable living. Eric's positive attitude and customer service–oriented approach were just as important to his success as the bacon. "In ten years, I sold almost 400 tons of potatoes. I sold tons and tons of bacon because bacon went on everything. We were real generous with the bacon. I charged more than anyone else, but I had the best quality product money could buy—even my ketchup and mustard were of higher quality. Everything was really clean, we dressed in uniforms, and we gained a level of trust with our customers to the point that people would bring their families down to see us all the time. We became the place people would come to from the airport—it would be the first place they'd go when they fly in at night. When I was starting to close up and get ready to retire, people were very upset." It was indeed a sad day in Boise when you could no longer get a 2:00 A.M. Chick Bacon on a Tater. The city lost a piece of its soul the day Eric Savage retired.

In 2007, about a year after Eric had retired and moved to Arizona, Boise State University's football team was playing in the Fiesta Bowl in Glendale, Arizona. Eric decided to set up a Chick Bacon on a Tater operation in the parking lot outside of the stadium. There were thousands of people there from Boise, and many of them could smell the familiar scent of the Chick Bacon on a Tater as they walked through the parking lot. "A lot of people came up to me and said, 'I knew it was you! I could smell the Chick Bacon on a Tater!' We had a huge crowd before the football game." There are a lot of bacon lovers in Idaho who pray that the Chick Bacon on a Tater will someday return to the streets of downtown Boise.

THE BACON NATION MEETS THE FAST-FOOD NATION

- **A&W** was the first restaurant chain to add bacon to a cheeseburger.

- **Sonic Drive-In** lets their customers add bacon to any of the sandwiches on their menu.

- In a typical year, **Cracker Barrel** serves 124 million slices of bacon.

- **Bojangles** serves breakfast all day long, and their menu has several items that include bacon (most notably the Bacon Biscuit).

- **The Original Pancake House** serves a Bacon Pancake, buttermilk pancakes filled with real bits of bacon.

- **Wendy's** serves a sandwich called The Baconator, which includes six strips of hickory-smoked bacon stacked with two quarter-pound hamburger patties. They have also featured the Big Bacon Classic on their menu in the past (a group of customers has launched an online petition urging Wendy's to put it back on the menu).

- **The Waffle House** has served 786,449,152 slices of bacon since 1955. If you lay all of the bacon end-to-end that Waffle House serves in a year, it will stretch from Atlanta to Los Angeles seven times.

SOME GUYS WHO REALLY LIKE BACON

Most frequent fliers will admit they have a weakness when it comes to how they spend their time at the airport. Some people can't resist the seductive aroma that emanates from Cinnabon. Others take refuge in the nearest cocktail lounge. For some of us, our weakness is meat-related.

Tucked away in a corner of Ronald Reagan Washington National Airport's Terminal C is an unusual slice of airport heaven called Five Guys Burgers and Fries. Five Guys is not the kind of food you would expect to encounter at an airport terminal (that is, it doesn't suck). Five Guys is a fast-food restaurant chain created in 1986 in nearby Arlington, Virginia, by Janie and Jerry Murrell and their five sons (hence the "Five Guys"). They started out with only one restaurant in a shopping center, but due to overwhelming popularity, opened more locations over the years and eventually franchised the store into more than 200 spots around the country. Millions of Americans are now able to experience the joy that is a Five Guys bacon cheeseburger.

Besides their delicious burgers, the other reason so many people on the East Coast are infatuated with Five Guys is their unabashed love of bacon.

Obviously the main offering at Five Guys is the hamburger. All of the burgers are offered with the additional options of cheese and bacon, along with an extensive selection of free toppings. But burgers aren't the only way you can get your bacon on. The menu also offers a hot dog with cheese and bacon. You might feel like you want to keel over and die right in the middle of the airport anytime you eat one of these creations—mostly because of the pure joy one experiences from consuming a Five Guys bacon cheese dog.

But it gets even better. One of the benefits of eating at the National

Airport location of Five Guys is that they are one of the few locations to serve breakfast. If you aren't a morning person, Five Guys can be your support system for surviving the airport during the early hours of the day. The main item on the breakfast menu is an egg sandwich that you can get with either a burger patty or bacon (or both if you are brave). They also offer the unusual option of a BLT sandwich for breakfast, just to make sure you have enough bacon options to satisfy your needs.

Bacon is such a prominent feature that at the National Airport Five Guys location there is always a basket of crispy bacon placed front and center on the prep table in plain view of customers and within arm's reach of any of the restaurant employees who are assembling the various sandwiches. And they burn through bacon like it's going out of style (which we all know will never happen).

Five Guys may have done their part to perfect the art of bacon burgers, but A&W Restaurants claim to be the first fast-food chain to put bacon on a cheeseburger. And thanks to pioneering bacon cheeseburger efforts, these days it's pretty difficult to find a fast-food restaurant, or any restaurant serving hamburgers for that matter, that doesn't offer bacon as a condiment option.

Another great chain restaurant for bacon hamburgers is Red Robin. One of their most popular burger options is the Royal Red Robin Burger—a hamburger topped with a fried egg, three strips of hickory-smoked bacon, American cheese, lettuce, tomatoes, and mayo. It's like the best of a bacon, egg, and cheese sandwich and a bacon cheeseburger all rolled into one. It's both efficient and tasty.

THE KENTUCKY HOT BROWN EXPERIENCE

If you ever find yourself in the lovely state of Kentucky, it's worth checking out one of the finer uses of bacon as a flavor enhancer, the **Kentucky Hot Brown**. Hot Brown sandwiches originated in Louisville, Kentucky, at the Brown Hotel in 1926. The hotel wanted to create a signature sandwich, and the Hot Brown was the result of that effort. The Hot Brown is an open-faced sandwich prepared by layering turkey, bacon, and Mornay sauce (a creamy white cheese sauce) on a slice of white bread. It's then broiled until the bread is crispy and the sauce begins to brown. Over the years its popularity has spread beyond Louisville throughout the rest of Kentucky, and while there are many local variations, a Hot Brown always revolves around these four basic ingredients.

Ramsey's Diner in Lexington is another great place to have a Hot Brown experience. The **Ramsey's Hot Brown** consists of (in order from bottom to top): white toast, sliced turkey, sliced ham, sliced tomatoes, Mornay sauce, Cheddar cheese, and two crispy slices of bacon. This gooey madness fills up an entire dinner plate and is far more than one person should consume in one sitting—it's best to share it with a friend (or two). The combination of flavors is comforting, pleasurable, and wicked all at once. And you'll probably want to start a new diet the following day.

BACON: THE BEST KEPT SECRET OF TOP RESTAURANTS

We've spent a lot of time here talking about the use of bacon as a flavor enhancer at fast-food and casual dining establishments. But chefs at fine dining restaurants are just as likely to use bacon as a secret weapon in the kitchen.

Todd Gray is the executive chef and co-owner of the award-winning restaurant Equinox in Washington, DC. Equinox is located mere steps from the White House, and they cater to dignitaries, celebrities, and famous (as well as infamous) Washingtonians on a daily basis. Despite their discriminating, upscale clientele, Chef Gray has absolutely no hesitation about using something as common as bacon in his kitchen.

The menu at Equinox focuses on the use of local, seasonal ingredients, but "bacon is always on the menu in some shape or form, all times of the year," according to Chef Gray. "Bacon is popular because of its diversity with respect to adding layers of flavor and in many senses seasoning a product. I like wrapping meats and fish in bacon and using lardons. With the exception of delicate white fish like Dover sole or turbot, almost everything can be paired with bacon." Once again, another top chef makes the point that everything is better with bacon (as if we didn't already know).

Like many chefs, Todd Gray also experiments with making his own bacon. "Many of us now make our own bacon with the help of small farmers producing heritage breeds of pork." Nothing says love more than house-made bacon.

Chef Dustan Bristol of Brick 29 bistro in Nampa, Idaho, is also reintroducing bacon in a whole new light to patrons of his restaurant. Nampa is a traditional town just west of Boise, and it's a place where very few restaurants that offer anything but meat and potatoes–style dining survive. But somehow Chef Bristol has managed to create one of the best dining experiences in Idaho. He is using bacon to help his customers bridge the gap between the down-home comfort foods most of them are familiar with, and the edgier, unique creations that are gaining him recognition as a highly talented chef.

One of the most popular items on the menu at Brick 29 is the B.L.A.T. (caramelized bacon, lettuce, avocado, and tomato on a crusty baguette). Yes, you read that correctly—caramelized bacon on a BLT sandwich. A traditional BLT is always enjoyable, but once you experience a B.L.A.T., a boring ol' BLT will never taste quite the same. For Chef Bristol, the B.L.A.T. just made a lot of sense to offer as an item on his menu. "I came up with the idea considering that the restaurant has an identity as a bistro, and I wanted to do something simple but delicious." And the inspiration behind this masterpiece? "Bacon." Of course.

Like many chefs, Dustan Bristol likes using bacon in his kitchen as a flavor enhancer. "Cooks love bacon!!! My philosophy is that 'fat is flavor' and Brick 29's trilogy is bacon, butter, and cream." The B.L.A.T. isn't the only bacon-blessed item on the Brick 29 menu. They also render bacon for use on salads, and they baste their steaks with bacon fat. Other ways Chef Bristol likes to cook with bacon are "risotto, pasta dishes, salads, and on a crusty baguette." You really can't escape the presence of bacon at Brick 29.

This author once hosted a dinner for family at Brick 29 and asked Chef Bristol to create a four-course meal in which cured pork made an appearance in every dish. He took the request, ran with it, and knocked the result out of the ballpark. The meal started with a Halloumi-style fried cheese topped with crispy prosciutto bits. Next was pumpkin bisque topped with bacon bits. The main course consisted of duck confit on a bed of creamed corn with bacon. Creamed corn is another sweet-tasting vegetable that goes really well with salty bacon. Our family was in hog heaven by the end of the meal.

LITTLE BITS O' BACON

In France, lardons are a popular bacon product. Also made from pork belly, lardons are fatty strips or cubes of bacon that are used to flavor stews, potato dishes, omelets, quiches, and as a topping for salads. *Frisée aux lardons* is a popular French salad that consists of a bed of frisée chicory leaves topped with lardons and a poached egg and drizzled with a vinegar-based dressing. This salad is a delicious classic, and fortunately it's increasingly making an appearance on the menus of restaurants throughout the United States. Next time you encounter frisée aux lardons at a restaurant, order it. It's a guaranteed form of *amour.*

David Lebovitz is a chef and author who lives in Paris. In France, he buys his bacon from a local charcuterie where one can typically purchase a gloriously wide variety of pork products. "They have a big slab and you tell them how much to cut, and how thick. It's called *poitrine fumée*—smoked belly. I get a thick slab and cut it into lardons or *bâtons* at home. It tastes really good and isn't pumped up with water like commercial bacon. It also doesn't exude any grease. When you cook it, you need to add oil to the pan, which is strange to Americans used to fatty bacon."

While most Americans might not be familiar with lardons, almost all of us are familiar with bacon bits. Very familiar. It's safe to say that 99 percent of restaurant salad bars have bacon bits as an option. You can also buy them by the bag at the grocery store if you want to have bacon bits on hand at home without having to go through the effort of frying the bacon yourself. When purchasing bacon bits to store in your refrigerator, it's best to focus on the real kind—not the imitation version that can be purchased in a bottle and kept in your spice cabinet for creepishly long periods of time (although many people do enjoy that version of bacon as a condiment). The bottom line is: we all like the idea of having bacon at our fingertips, and there are a lot of ways to accomplish that goal.

The uses for bacon bits are truly unlimited. Sprinkling them on a salad is probably the most common one. A fresh wedge of lettuce dressed with creamy blue cheese and topped with bacon bits is not only an easy salad to make but it's also quite refreshing and perfect for a hot summer day. Another typical way to eat bacon bits is to sprinkle them on a baked potato. Don't you love when you order a baked potato at a restaurant and they bring that tower of condiment options to the table and ask if you would like sour cream, butter, chives, *or* bacon bits? Any rational person would reply with "Load me up!" Why should we have to choose between those options when we can have them all? But if forced to make a choice, it's pretty obvious that bacon bits would win.

Bacon bits are also good sprinkled on clam chowder or any other cream-based soup. Or they can be used in cooking to flavor a dish if you don't have easy access to lardons or fresh crumbled bacon. Spaghetti carbonara is a classic dish in which bacon plays a starring role, and if you always have bacon bits on hand, you can throw this Italian pasta dish together in no time.

More than anything, what's great about bacon bits is the idea of bacon as a standard condiment and something that you can sprinkle on almost any food, just like salt or pepper. It's another one of those uses for bacon that sometimes makes you wonder who the first person was to come up with the idea. It's as if bacon for breakfast just wasn't enough; at some point, some genius decided that humans needed a means for consuming bacon throughout the day without just constantly frying and eating individual strips of it. And the solution was to fry some extra bacon, crumble it into bits, and set it aside to put on top of anything else we eat. With such versatility and abundance, it really is no wonder that bacon is such a big part of our food culture.

BACON AND BLEU SALAD

Bacon and bleu salad is one of Chef Greggory Hill's favorite things to eat. Enjoy it with a bottle of Shiraz.

SERVES 4

FOR THE DRESSING

1 cup mayonnaise
½ cup sour cream
¼ cup buttermilk
2 teaspoons Tabasco sauce
1 clove garlic, chopped
2 tablespoons chopped green onion (scallion)
1 cup crumbled creamy blue cheese (¼ pound)
1 teaspoon kosher salt

FOR THE SALAD

8 slices of your favorite bacon
1 head iceberg lettuce
1 large red bell pepper, roasted, cooled, peeled, and seeded
½ cup creamy blue cheese (2 ounces)
Sea salt and cracked black pepper

1. Cook the bacon in a cast-iron skillet or in a 350°F oven for 8 to 10 minutes, until crisp. Remove the bacon and place on a paper towel–lined plate. Reserve the bacon fat for the dressing and let cool slightly.

2. To make the dressing, combine 6 tablespoons of the bacon drippings with the mayonnaise, sour cream, buttermilk, Tabasco, garlic, green onion, blue cheese, and salt in a food processor and mix until incorporated. Transfer to a covered container and refrigerate until needed.

3. To make the salad, cut the lettuce into four wedges. Cut the roasted pepper into thin strips. Place 2 to 3 tablespoons of dressing in the center of each of four salad plates. Place a wedge of lettuce on top of the dressing. Divide the remaining dressing over the lettuce wedges. Drape the roasted pepper strips over the wedges. Place 2 strips of bacon into each of the wedges between the leaves. Crumble the blue cheese over the salads. Season with sea salt and cracked black pepper. Serve immediately.

BLACK PEPPER BACON CHILI

This chili goes well with beer or wine. Enjoy the fruits of your labor while watching the Super Bowl or just on a cold February evening.

SERVES 12 TO 15

1 pound dried pinto beans
1 pound dried black beans
Low-sodium beef broth
8 dried ancho chiles, stemmed, seeded, soaked in hot water until soft, and drained
¼ cup olive oil
3 medium white onions, cut into small dice
3 cloves garlic, minced
½ pound black pepper bacon, cut into ½-inch pieces
3 tablespoons ground cumin

1 orange, scrubbed and cut in half
2 tablespoons kosher salt
2 bay leaves
15 tomatoes, seeded and cut into medium dice
1 tablespoon fresh chopped oregano
3 tablespoons fresh chopped cilantro

1. Pick over and rinse the pinto and black beans. Place in a large container, cover with cold water by several inches, and soak overnight.
2. The next day drain the beans, and place them in a large saucepan. Cover with half water and half beef broth by at least 3 inches. Bring to a boil over high heat, then lower to a simmer. Cook for about 40 minutes, until the beans are almost tender.
3. Cut open the ancho chiles and scrape out the flesh (discard the skins). Heat the olive oil in a stockpot over medium heat. Add the onions, garlic, and chile paste. Sauté, stirring frequently, until the onions are translucent.
4. Add the bacon and cook until the fat starts to render out. Add the cumin, orange, salt, bay leaves, tomatoes, and the beans along with their cooking liquid. Cook for 30 minutes more.
5. Add the oregano and cilantro. Cook until the beans are tender and the mixture has thickened. Remove the bay leaves and orange halves before serving.
6. Serve with white rice and grated Cheddar cheese, if you choose.

BEEF AND BACON STROGANOFF

Beef Stroganoff is a delicious, comfort food, and it is very quick and easy to prepare after a long day at work. Naturally, it is even better when you add bacon.

SERVES 4

6 slices hickory-smoked bacon, cut into ½-inch pieces
1½ pounds beef, cut into 1-inch cubes (use a tender cut that will cook quickly)
3 large white mushrooms, trimmed, wiped clean, and cut into medium dice
One 10.75-ounce can of Campbell's Condensed Cream of Mushroom soup
½ cup water
1 tablespoon Worcestershire sauce
8 ounces egg noodles

1. Bring a large pot of salted water to a boil.

2. While the water for the noodles is heating, cook the bacon until crispy in a large skillet over medium heat. Remove the bacon with a slotted spoon to a paper towel–lined plate. Leave the bacon drippings in the skillet.

3. Add the beef to the drippings and brown on all sides over medium heat. Cook only until the centers are medium rare.

4. Add the mushrooms to the skillet and sauté for 3 minutes. Stir in the soup, water, and Worcestershire sauce. Add the bacon and mix together well. Simmer over low heat for 10 minutes.

5. When the water boils, cook the egg noodles according to the package directions. When the noodles are done, drain them in a colander.

6. Divide the noodles among four serving bowls. Top with the beef and sauce and serve immediately.

BACON AND CHICKEN QUESADILLAS WITH GUACAMOLE AND SOUR CREAM

How can you not get in a festive mood with some delicious quesadillas?
Add bacon to the mix and it's a party you'll never forget.

SERVES 6 TO 8

FOR THE GUACAMOLE

3 avocados, preferably Hass
Juice of 1 lime
1 tablespoon kosher salt
1 small red onion, cut into small dice
1 bunch cilantro, chopped
1 serrano chile, stemmed, seeded if you prefer it less spicy, and cut into small dice
1 tomato, seeded and cut into small dice

FOR THE QUESADILLAS

1 pound bacon (your favorite), cut into 1-inch pieces
Four 4-ounce chicken breast halves
2 tablespoons ground cumin
2 tablespoons ground coriander
1 tablespoon kosher salt
3 ounces grated white Cheddar cheese
3 ounces grated Monterey Jack cheese
3 ounces grated pepper Jack cheese
2 tablespoons chopped cilantro
2 tablespoons chopped green onion (scallion)
Eight 8-inch flour tortillas
Sour cream, for serving
Lime wedges, for serving
Cilantro sprigs, for serving

1. To make the guacamole, cut the avocados in half and remove the pits. Scoop the flesh into a medium bowl. Add the lime juice and salt and mash the avocado as much as you like, anywhere from totally smooth to fairly chunky. Fold in the onion, cilantro, chile, and tomato. Cover with plastic wrap directly on the surface and refrigerate until needed.

2. To make the quesadillas, preheat the oven to 350°F. In a large ovenproof cast-iron skillet over medium heat, cook the bacon until crispy. Remove the bacon with a slotted spoon to a paper towel–lined plate. Carefully pour half the bacon fat into a heatproof container; leave the rest in the skillet.

3. Put the chicken in a large bowl. Pour about ¼ cup of the reserved bacon fat over the chicken breasts and toss to coat. In a small bowl, mix the cumin, coriander, and salt. Sprinkle the spices over the chicken breasts and toss to coat.

4. Heat the skillet again over medium heat. Add the chicken pieces to the fat in the skillet and cook for 4 minutes. Turn over and cook for another 4 minutes. Place the skillet in the oven for 8 to 10 minutes to finish cooking the chicken.

5. Remove the skillet from the oven and transfer the chicken to a plate to cool. Leave the oven on. When the chicken is cool enough to handle, slice in half, then cut lengthwise into strips. Set aside. Wipe out the skillet.

6. In a medium bowl, mix together the three cheeses. In a small bowl, mix together the cilantro and green onion.

7. Return the skillet to medium heat. One at a time, brush a tortilla on both sides with the reserved bacon fat and place it in the skillet. Heat for 2 minutes on one side, then turn over. Place about 2 tablespoons of the cheese mixture on the tortilla, then some

bacon, chicken, and herbs. Fold the tortilla over and turn until the cheese is melted. Place on a baking sheet in the oven to keep warm. Continue with the remaining tortillas, cheese, bacon, chicken, and herbs.

8. To serve, top with the guacamole and a dollop of sour cream, and garnish with a lime wedge and a cilantro sprig.

MACARONI AND CHEESE WITH BACON

Mac 'n' cheese isn't just for kids anymore. This bacon-blessed version is sure to please anyone with a pulse. This recipe is courtesy of Dennis, a Los Angeles–based bacon fanatic.

SERVES 2 TO 3

2 cups uncooked orecchiette or farfalle pasta
2 tablespoons (¼ stick) unsalted butter
1 teaspoon salt
½ teaspoon ground black pepper
⅓ cup all-purpose flour
¾ cup heavy cream
½ cup plain yogurt
1 cup crumbled blue cheese
½ cup grated Parmesan cheese
3 to 4 slices crisply fried bacon, crumbled

1. Bring a large pot of salted water to a boil and cook the pasta al dente. Drain in a colander and keep warm.
2. Melt the butter in a large saucepan over medium heat. Stir in the

salt, black pepper, and flour and cook, stirring frequently, until the flour just begins to color. Stir in the cream and cook until the mixture thickens slightly. Stir in the yogurt, blue cheese, and Parmesan until the cheeses are melted. Stir in the bacon and pasta and cook just until everything is hot. Serve immediately.

CHAPTER 9

THE MAIN COURSE–STARRING BACON, THE BEST MEAT EVER

"Life expectancy would grow by leaps and bounds if green vegetables smelled as good as bacon."
—DOUG LARSON

DESPITE HOW MUCH people love bacon, many still think of it as a food that should be served on the side at breakfast or as a flavor enhancer to make something else taste better. But consumers are finally warming up to the idea that it doesn't have to be just a side dish or a condiment. Bacon can, indeed, be the main feature of a meal, and it plays the starring role admirably when given the opportunity.

Truth be told, bacon is far more versatile than most of us realize. Slices might turn up layered between the leaves of a wedge of lettuce, and the dressing might feature bacon as the central flavor ingredient. Bacon as the main topping for a pizza is becoming more common—most of the major pizza chains now offer it, beyond the traditional Canadian bacon option. Bacon is the primary meat in numerous pasta sauces—and leftover bacon grease can serve as a flavorful foundation to hold the sauce together. And let us not forget to praise that all-American classic, the BLT. With such abundant versatility in mind, it should come as no surprise that bacon's status in kitchens across the country has enjoyed a metamorphosis in recent years. It is no longer considered an afterthought or accompaniment by the nation's top chefs. In fact, bacon now rules the menus of many fine dining establishments. And patrons of those restaurants are embracing the increased availability of bacon wholeheartedly.

The act of enjoying a single slice of bacon is nothing new. Pork cures just about better than most any other meat, which is what led to its popularity prior to the invention of modern-day refrigeration. Ancient Greeks and Romans were known for their indulgent extracurricular activities such as eating for pleasure, and they enjoyed salted pork quite regularly. The Romans fed pigs figs and honey to enhance the flavor of the meat, and then they prepared shoulder bacon for consumption by browning it—similar to the way we fry bacon today. Bacon was also a prominent part of the Anglo-Saxon diet. Our affinity for bacon is practically ingrained in our DNA.

A HEALTHY BACON OBSESSION

A previous chapter introduced you to Chef Greggory Hill, whose restaurant David Greggory in Washington, DC, was for several years a haven for the Bacon Nation. Between his weekly Pork and Pinot Happy Hours, monthly Aphrodisiac Bacon Dinners, and the regular restaurant menu, bacon lovers in our nation's capital could indulge excessively in The Best Meat Ever whenever they felt the urge, and they could do it in a friendly environment where no one would judge their obsession. No other chef in the United States embraces the concept of bacon as the main event better than Chef Hill. It was seriously depressing the day his restaurant changed ownership and the bacon-friendly format rode off into the sunset.

Chef Hill's love for bacon began at an early age. "When I was a child, at my aunt and uncle's house, they always had pigs. We always had the jar of pig fat that the eggs got cooked in and the bread got dipped in. I was always around it and it just became a big part of the flavor component of a lot of my food. I've just always been around it and I like it." Maybe Chef Hill's love of bacon wasn't genetic, but it was most certainly a product of his environment.

To create entire menus around bacon, it is necessary to experiment with many bacon varieties. Chef Hill, like most other chefs around the country, embraces artisanal bacons for his many needs. "There are a lot of artisanal bacons out there . . . it's amazing. Especially when you have the luxury of having ten or twelve of them in the house at the same time and you get to taste the difference." Wow, what a rough job—having to taste several kinds of bacon every day. Don't you feel bad for him?

To come up with all of his unique bacon creations, Chef Hill eats far more bacon than the average person does on a daily basis, and probably even more than most other chefs. But he still has some favorite dishes that he could eat every day, and amazingly he never gets sick of bacon. "I could just eat a bowl of bacon. I eat bacon every day. I could eat it all the time with blue cheese and iceberg lettuce. Pork chops. Macaroni and cheese with bacon fat. And the BLT. I really loved our BLT." If the Bacon Nation were to have a leader, Chef Hill would be an ideal candidate for the job.

BACON APPETIZERS

Not surprisingly, bacon has also crept onto the appetizer menus of restaurants across the United States. And good fortune for all of us that it has! Bacon as appetizer . . . it's so simple that it's brilliant—why not get your meal off to a roaring start with a big ol' side of bacon? Talk about setting a good tone for the rest of the meal.

Even though the idea of bacon on its own as an appetizer seems so simple, there are actually several different ways to execute the concept. At Psycho Suzi's Motor Lounge, a tiki-themed restaurant in Minneapolis, Minnesota, the Plate 'o Bacon appetizer is merely a plate of applewood-smoked bacon slices wrapped into curls and individually skewered with toothpicks. It's the perfect dish to share with friends, and fortunately the toothpicks aren't sharp enough to do too much damage as you're fighting each other for the last piece. Across town from Psycho Suzi's is an upscale steakhouse called Manny's. The bacon starter there is somewhat "meatier"—their bacon is served as two chunks (for lack of a better word) of very thick applewood-smoked bacon that has been grilled so that the edges are crispy but the center is still chewy and rich with luscious strips of fat. It's far more than one person should eat in one sitting, especially if you're planning to also have a steak for dinner. It could easily be the main event itself.

Minneapolis isn't the only town where you can kick off your meal with bacon. Another steakhouse well known for its bacon appetizer is BLT Steak, which has outposts in New York City, Washington, DC, and a few other large cities across the United States. BLT doesn't stand for the sandwich of the same name—it actually stands for Bistro Laurent Tourondel. Tourondel is the restaurant's executive chef. But even though the BLT name can be misleading for those of us who are singularly focused on all things porcine, the bacon appetizer at BLT Steak is no joke. Its double-cut bacon is served with a vinegar and garlic dressing, and best avoided if you have a weak palate. Peter Luger Steakhouse in Brooklyn, New York, also follows in the steakhouse tradition of offering a bacon appetizer. Their version is a large, sizzling slice of extra-thick bacon to whet your appetite for more meat (or curb your appetite, depending on the size of your stomach).

The concept of bacon as an appetizer or stand-alone dish isn't anything new. It's simply an American twist on the European concept called *charcuterie* (French) or *salumi* (Italian), which are the broad terms used for the school of cooking that involves curing meats. These words are now commonly used to describe an item on restaurant menus that is simply a plate of cured meats.

TO CURE OR NOT TO CURE

Most people are familiar with pork belly only because they've eaten it cured as bacon. But when properly prepared, uncured pork belly is one of the most enjoyable culinary delights in this world. The most common way to prepare uncured pork belly is to braise it, which creates scrumptious strips of velvety fat layered between juicy slices of meat with a crispy outside. It's enough to make you drool just thinking about it.

THE ALL-YOU-CAN-EAT BACON SENSATION SWEEPING THE NATION

There are countless dining establishments in the United States capitalizing on bacon's current popularity. Many bars and restaurants have recognized its power, and they are featuring all-you-can-eat bacon events to attract customers to their business. There is no better way to feature bacon as the main event than a bottomless basket of it!

Tuesday night is Bacon Night at the Harris Grill in Pittsburgh, Pennsylvania. Harris Grill was one of the first restaurants in the country to feature an all-you-can-eat bacon event. On an all-you-can-eat night, you can have free bacon at the bar from happy hour until the bar closes (or "until the pigs go home," as the staff likes to say), and people sitting at tables can get their bacon fix for just one dollar. Either way, it's a good deal. The restaurant closed for a few months in late 2007 due to a fire, but it's open again and serving bacon with a vengeance.

In Chicago, a bar called Whiskey Road features all-you-can-eat bacon for ten dollars every Monday. Talk about a good way to start the work week.

The Godspeed Café in Oakland, California, serves all-you-can-eat waffles, bacon, and mimosas on Saturday morning for seven dollars.

This restaurant is actually connected to a motor bike shop, and they have a tattoo parlor. Waffles, bacon, motorized vehicles, tattoos, and booze on a Saturday morning . . . sounds like a recipe for a lot of fun (or a lot of trouble).

The Triple Rock Social Club in Minneapolis, Minnesota, is a popular place to go for live music, but on Wednesdays bacon is the star attraction. Free Bacon Wednesdays offer all-you-can-eat bacon from 9:00 to 11:00 P.M. or until the bacon runs out.

Of course, you don't need a bar or restaurant in your hometown with a specific all-you-can-eat bacon offering to experience the joy of eating as much bacon as you can before you explode. Most all-you-can-eat buffet restaurants that can be found in any corner of the United States offer bacon as an option, and these restaurants usually allow you to eat an infinite amount of bacon along with anything else your heart desires, for a reasonable price. So if you don't live in Pittsburgh, Chicago, Oakland, or any other town with a dedicated bottomless bacon event, create your own all-you-can-eat bacon event at your favorite local feeding trough. Take a group of friends and make it a party. Do bacon proud and make a showing that results in the restaurant rethinking its all-you-can-eat policy.

HOUSE BACON

Another trend in the restaurant industry that is gaining in popularity is the art of curing bacon in-house. Despite the increasing availability of artisanal bacons, some restaurants want total control over the quality and taste of the bacon they serve. They also want to create bacon that fits the specific needs of their menu. It is no longer unusual to walk into the refrigerator of an upscale restaurant and find anywhere from one to several experimental slabs being cured using a variety of methods and flavors. And there's something comforting about knowing there is a slab of bacon curing mere steps from where you are enjoying a bacon-blessed entrée.

EatBar and Tallula are sister restaurants in Arlington, Virginia, that are bastions of porcine goodness, and the house-cured bacon is one of the most popular items on the menu at both establishments. It isn't unusual for their house bacon to be sold out, leaving their patrons hungry for more and sure to return for another bite at the apple. Or, in this case, pig. Taking a gastropub approach to their menu, almost all of their cured meats are produced onsite. In 2007, during the Chinese Year of the Pig, Chef Nathan Anda got the idea to add a "bacon of the week" to his menu of house-made charcuterie. But Chef Anda doesn't make just any kind of bacon. Many of his bacons are infused with unusual flavors such as juniper, ginger, chocolate, star anise, cumin, coriander, cayenne, and vanilla. Old Bay is a popular seasoning to put on foods in East Coast states due to the availability of fresh seafood, so Chef Anda has experimented with it as a bacon flavor. He has also produced a coffee-flavored bacon to pair with doughnuts—a modern twist on a classic breakfast combination. He is definitely not afraid to push the boundaries of the flavored bacon movement, bless his experimental soul.

Despite the unusual flavors he plays with, Chef Anda takes a pretty traditional approach to curing his bacon. For his house bacon, he uses kosher salt, brown sugar, thyme, and garlic powder. He cures it for two weeks under refrigeration, then wipes off the cure and hangs it for three days. The bacon is then smoked in a mixture of mesquite and applewood. Perfectly simple and perfectly delicious.

Between EatBar and Tallula, Chef Anda's bacon finds its way onto the menu in a variety of ways. "We use the scraps of our house-cured bacon and grind them into bacon bits and use them as a garnish on salads. We wrap bacon around Mission figs and roast them." The house-made bacon at EatBar and Tallula isn't just a gimmicky promotional item—it truly is an integral part of the menu.

"I love to add bacon for depth of flavor, whether it is a meaty or smoky flavor or because the dish just needs some added fattiness. You can get so much out of bacon. You can render it down and just use its fat, you can wrap it around stuff to add moisture—it has endless possibilities." And it is endlessly delicious.

BACON THROUGHOUT HISTORY

- The Chinese were reportedly the first humans to domesticate pigs around 4300 B.C.

- In ancient Greece, browning a slice of shoulder bacon was a popular indulgence.

- The word "bacon" came into existence during the Middle Ages, initially to describe pork in general, and then later to describe cured pork belly specifically.

- Hogs were often onboard during voyages across the ocean from Europe to the New World. Those sailors had continual access to delicious pork products, which almost certainly gave them inspiration to keep traveling farther!

- The art of curing bacon has been handed down through generations, particularly in Missouri, Kentucky, and Tennessee. There you can find dozens of country-style smokehouses using methods based on the way bacon has been cured for hundreds of years.

- The BLT (bacon, lettuce, and tomato sandwich) became popular when fresh lettuce and tomatoes became available year-round with the rapid expansion of supermarkets after World War II.

Chef Anda believes that our affinity for bacon stems from our experiences with it in our youth. "People grew up eating it and have such fond memories of what it means to them. I think people love to talk about things that bring them back in time and bacon seems to have been a staple on a lot of people's breakfast tables. I used to love it when my mom cooked bacon in her cast-iron pan and then would let the fat congeal in the pan when she was done. I never needed butter." Bacon truly is the meat that keeps on giving.

BACON, ITALIAN STYLE

Mio Restaurant in downtown Washington, DC, is also embracing the art of curing their own meats. Chef Stefano Frigerio was born and raised in Inverigo, a small village in northern Italy. Chef Frigerio learned to cook from his grandmother, who he prepared family meals with side by side. "When I was a kid, my grandmother used to make her own salami. We would go to the farmers, get part of a belly or shoulder, we'd cure it, and then we'd grind it. That's where I learned to make salami." And the fascination (some might say obsession) with curing meats only grew from there.

Chef Frigerio's exposure to fresh ingredients and his grandmother's homemade salami naturally led to an interest in curing other meats. "With time, I started to experiment with pancetta. The first time it was a guess—I looked at the belly, sprinkled some salt on it, and let it cure for a couple of weeks. When I took it out, it was too salty. So I hung it to dry. Then we sliced it and it was still too salty. So I cured the next one for only a week, added more water, and continued to experiment with it." Practice makes perfect.

Chef Frigerio has been able to continue experimenting with the art of curing meats at his various positions in distinguished kitchens over the years, but at Mio he is able to incorporate more of his classic European culinary techniques into the daily menu.

"We are currently curing our own lardo, pancetta, guanciale, and prosciutto, in addition to marinating meat for salami. Pancetta is used mostly as a cooking garnish. We use it to flavor mushrooms, meats, and fish. Our lardo is used for cooking—for sauces and roasting meat. Our prosciutto can be served as a single dish by itself."

The pigs that Chef Frigerio uses for his cured meats come from a couple of local farmers and are either Ossabaw or Berkshire hogs. "The Ossabaws are smaller and fattier, and the Berkshires are bigger and darker in meat color." And these choice meats result in a choice of scrumptious cured meats for Mio customers.

Chef Frigerio likes the extra flavor he gets from curing his own meats. "Usually when I buy it, it's good, but it's nothing special—it doesn't satisfy me enough. If you go through the process to cure it yourself, and then you cook with it, you can taste big flavors inside the dish and you know where everything came from. Many dishes on our menu need a kick, and cured meat is a good way to do that."

As for whether Chef Frigerio prefers American-style bacon or Italian-style pancetta, the answer is pretty obvious given his Italian roots and cooking style. "I prefer pancetta. Bacon is good if you just sear it, but to incorporate it into long cooking, bacon releases the flavor very quickly and you lose it very quickly. Pancetta releases its flavor slower over a longer period of time and keeps the flavor longer. But with a couple of eggs, bacon is good." Despite the cultural differences, we can all agree with Chef Frigerio that cured pork belly is *delizioso*.

Clearly, Italians have been mastering the art of cured pork products for hundreds of years. Traditionally, the curing of meats was dictated by the seasons—pigs were fattened in summer and fall, and then slaughtered right before winter arrived. Pancetta is the Italian cured meat product most similar to American bacon. Also produced from pork belly, pancetta is salt cured and flavored with a variety of spices, but unlike American bacon, pancetta isn't smoked. The French also have their own version of pancetta called *ventrèche*.

A cousin of pancetta is prosciutto, which comes dry-cured and uncooked. Both products come from the pig and are cured, but prosciutto is actually ham, and therefore isn't considered to be part of the bacon family in the way that pancetta is (but we still love prosciutto anyway).

Recognizing that there was a shortage of high-quality Italian-style cured meats being produced commercially in the United States, Herb and Kathy Eckhouse started a company called La Quercia just outside of Des Moines, Iowa, in 2001. After living in the Parma region of Italy for three years while Herb was working for a seed company, the Eckhouses returned to Iowa with an appreciation for Parma's cured meats. They had seen how important cured meats are to the culture there, so they decided to try their hand at making those same meats back home. The timing was right in the late 1990s when Herb's employer was bought out and he made the decision to start his own business rather than find another job.

The Eckhouses started out by spending about five months studying prosciutto and deciding whether or not it would make sense to make it in Iowa. They had been told many times that the key to good prosciutto was the climate—something that would be difficult to replicate outside of Italy. They came to the conclusion that this was more legend than fact, however, and because of their ready access to pork from Iowa, the odds were in their favor.

Even though La Quercia started out by making prosciutto, the Eckhouses looked at pancetta early on. According to Herb, "Touring plants in Italy and seeing how pancetta was made, and seeing how we were set up, we figured we could make pancetta." And an Italian-style legacy in the American heartland was born.

La Quercia gets their meat from a few different producers in the Midwest, all of which use celebrated organic methods and raise their hogs in an antibiotic-free environment. "We have a basic screen which is no confinement, no subtherapeutic antibiotics, and no animal by-products in the feed. Within that we have our breed preferences, but we don't always get the breeds we prefer. Berkshire is our preference. Then we have a list of quality criteria for specific cuts—size, fat cover, color, and defects. We pay over commodity price—we pay a premium—because we want to be able to carry through those traits on the label." And La Quercia's products are definitely premium—they make some of the best Italian-style cured meats you'll ever get your paws on.

The La Quercia plant features state-of-the-art technology to replicate the climate for curing Italian-style meats that was traditionally environmental. "We worked with a guy from Italy to design the rooms. All the equipment comes from Italy."

"We generally work with three cuts: hams, bellies, and jowls. We make prosciutto, pancetta, and guanciale. We don't use any nitrates or nitrites because I think it's bad eating. I don't like the way they leave a tingling in my mouth or a burning in my throat."

La Quercia pancetta contains three basic, very traditional ingredients—pork, sea salt, and spices. For the spices they use juniper berry, bay leaf, black pepper, and white pepper. Pancetta made in Italy sometimes has garlic in it, but La Quercia doesn't use garlic. They sell both rolled and flat pancetta. "Rolled pancetta is easier for most American consumers to relate to. Because flat pancetta [is often eaten uncooked], they get scared because they think they're supposed to cook their bacon." And no one should ever be scared of bacon, that's for sure!

"We select our bellies relatively thick. It works well with our suppliers because they need the leaner bellies for bacon. We take the fat bellies because they're great for pancetta. It makes a product with a real creamy fat that just melts." La Quercia's melt-in-your-mouth pancetta will melt your heart.

The pancetta cures for about a month, which is about twice as long as most American-style bacon. The guanciale that La Quercia makes from pork jowls is cured similar to the way they cure the pancetta. They also make a lardo which is cured pork back fat (and is amazing when you melt it on a piece of toast—once you try it, you'll forget butter ever existed and will never want anything but lardo on your toast ever again).

So why the name La Quercia for the business? "La Quercia means 'the oak' in Italian. The oak is ubiquitous with the region Parma where we lived in Italy. It's a long-term association. It's also the state tree of Iowa." So it seems there are a lot of reasons why Herb and Kathy Eckhouse have been so successful with their Italian-style cured meats made in the heartland of America. More than anything, they are ensuring that more Americans have access to foods like pancetta, the notable relative of The Best Meat Ever.

RECIPES TO SATISFY YOUR BACON OBSESSION

A REFRESHING SUMMER BLT

BLTs are a great sandwich any time of year, but they are particularly good in late summer when you can make them with the freshest, juiciest tomatoes. The arugula spices up this sandwich with peppery flavor.

SERVES 1

2 to 3 strips thick-cut applewood-smoked bacon
2 slices sourdough bread
1 tablespoon mayonnaise or aïoli
3 to 4 arugula leaves
2 slices fresh buffalo mozzarella cheese
2 slices heirloom tomatoes

In a cast-iron skillet, cook the bacon to your desired level of crispiness. Toast the sourdough bread. Spread mayonnaise on each slice of bread. Stack the bacon, arugula, mozzarella, and tomatoes on one slice of bread, top with the other slice of bread and eat while the bread and bacon are still warm.

B.L.A.T. SANDWICH

Chef Dustan Bristol serves this sandwich at his restaurant Brick 29 in Nampa, Idaho. You have not had a BLT sandwich until you have had one made with caramelized bacon. If you have an addictive personality, you might want to seriously think twice before going down this path.

1 crusty baguette, sliced in half lengthwise
Mayonnaise
6 to 8 slices Caramelized Bacon, warm (recipe follows)
1 Hass avocado, pitted, peeled, and sliced thin
Boston or Bibb lettuce leaves, rinsed and dried
1 large tomato, sliced thin

If you like, lightly toast the baguette. Spread mayonnaise on the cut sides. On the bottom half, stack the bacon, avocado, lettuce, and tomato. Cover with the top half of the bread, press down lightly to mingle the goodness, and cut into four portions.

CARAMELIZED BACON

1 pound applewood-smoked thick-sliced bacon
½ cup packed dark brown sugar
2 tablespoon red pepper flakes

Preheat the oven to 350°F. Line a rimmed baking sheet with parchment paper. Lay out the bacon flat on the parchment. Sprinkle with the brown sugar in an even layer. Sprinkle with the red pepper flakes. Bake until crispy, 15 to 18 minutes. Let the bacon cool in the pan for a couple of minutes so the sugar can caramelize. This can be made in advance and reheated in the oven for a couple of minutes.

SPAGHETTI CARBONARA

Carbonara is a classic Italian pasta dish. It was traditionally made with guanciale or pancetta, but American bacon has a heavier smoky flavor that really makes bacon the focal point of this dish.

SERVES 4

½ pound bacon
8 ounces spaghetti
4 large eggs
Salt
Freshly ground black pepper
Grated Parmesan cheese

1. In a large cast-iron or other heavy skillet, cook the bacon over medium heat until crispy. Remove the bacon and place it on a paper towel–lined plate. Reserve the bacon grease in the skillet. Once the bacon has cooled enough to touch, crumble it into small pieces.
2. Meanwhile, bring a large pot of salted water to a boil. Cook the spaghetti al dente, according to the package directions. Drain in a colander and return the spaghetti to the pot over low heat. Spoon 3 tablespoons of the bacon fat into the pot and add the bacon. Mix together.
3. Whisk the eggs in a small bowl until blended. Add salt to taste.
4. Remove the pot from the heat and add the eggs. Stir quickly for 30 seconds. Season with black pepper and serve immediately, sprinkled with Parmesan cheese.

HUNGARIAN RICE

This recipe comes courtesy of a Bacon Unwrapped reader named Steph: "Our standby bacon-based entrée is what my husband calls Hungarian Rice." This dish is a perfect example of how the use of bacon and a few simple ingredients can make an incredibly delicious entrée.

SERVES 4 TO 6

1 pound sliced bacon (your favorite)
2 cloves garlic, finely minced
4 cups cooked rice (your choice)
1 cup frozen peas, thawed and drained
Salt and pepper

1. In a large cast-iron or other heavy skillet, cook the bacon over medium heat until crispy. Remove the bacon and place it on a paper towel–lined plate. Reserve the bacon grease in the skillet. Once the bacon has cooled enough to touch, chop it coarsely.

2. Add the garlic to the drippings in the skillet and cook over medium heat just enough to bring out the flavor. Add the rice and heat, stirring to get the drippings and garlic mixed in well. Add the bacon and peas. Continue cooking until the peas are heated through. Add salt and pepper to taste. Serve hot.

JALAPEÑO-BACON PIZZA

Bacon pizza is becoming increasingly popular, and adding jalapeños gives it an exciting spicy kick. If you can find jalapeño-flavored bacon, even better. The dough recipe can also be used to make a breakfast pizza topped with bacon, eggs, and cheese. This recipe is courtesy of Rocco Loosbrock and Brenda Beaman of Coastal Vineyards.

SERVES 12

DOUGH

¾ cup warm water (about 110°F)
One ¼-ounce packet (2¼ teaspoons) active dry yeast
   (not instant or quick-rise)
2½ teaspoons sugar
½ teaspoon kosher salt
1 cup whole wheat flour
½ cup all-purpose flour, plus extra for kneading (optional)
Nonstick cooking spray

SAUCE

1 cup tomato sauce
6 tablespoons (half of a 6-ounce can) tomato paste
1 teaspoon dried Mexican oregano
¼ teaspoon kosher salt

PICO DE GALLO

1½ cups seeded and diced tomatoes (if you have to use
   canned, drain before measuring)
½ cup diced white onions (about half of a medium onion)

1 tablespoon minced cilantro
1 clove garlic, finely grated
½ teaspoon kosher salt

TOPPINGS

¾ pound bacon, cut into ½-inch pieces
¾ cup crumbled queso fresco
Shredded lettuce
¼ cup sour cream
1 large fresh jalapeño chile, stemmed, seeded if you prefer
    less spice, and cut into 12 slices

1. Combine the water, yeast, and sugar in the bowl of a stand mixer. Let sit about 5 minutes for the yeast to begin bubbling. Add the salt and whole wheat flour and beat on medium speed with a whip attachment for 3 minutes to develop the gluten.

2. Remove the whip and attach the dough hook. Add the all-purpose flour and mix, starting slowly until most of the flour has been incorporated. Knead the dough on medium speed for 3 minutes. Remove the dough hook and cover the bowl loosely with plastic wrap. Allow the dough to rise at room temperature until it has about doubled, 45 minutes to 1 hour. (If you don't have a dough hook for your mixer, stir in the all-purpose flour with a sturdy spoon. Dump the dough out onto a lightly floured work surface and knead by hand until the dough holds together and is smooth and elastic. Spray a large bowl with nonstick cooking spray, put the dough in, cover with plastic wrap, and let it rise until doubled.)

3. While the dough is rising, prepare the sauce and toppings. Stir together the tomato sauce, tomato paste, oregano, and salt for the pizza sauce in a small bowl and set aside. Combine the tomatoes, onions, cilantro, garlic, and salt for the pico de gallo in a medium bowl. Transfer to a fine-mesh strainer and allow it to drain over a bowl for at least 10 minutes.

4. Fry the bacon in a cast-iron or other heavy skillet over medium-high heat, stirring occasionally for even browning. When the bacon is cooked to your desired doneness, remove the bacon with a slotted spoon to a paper towel–lined plate. Once the bacon is cool enough to touch, shred it into bite-size pieces.

5. Preheat the oven to 500°F. Spray a small area of a clean countertop with nonstick cooking spray. Flatten and shape the dough into a 14-inch circle. Liberally spray the dough with nonstick cooking spray to ensure easy release from the pan. Flip the dough over onto a 14-inch pizza pan.

6. Spread about ⅔ cup of the pizza sauce onto the dough. (Use more or less depending on your taste.) Sprinkle all but ½ cup of the bacon and ⅓ cup of the queso fresco evenly over the pizza. Bake the pizza for about 7 minutes, until the crust is golden brown on the edges. Remove the pizza from the oven and let cool for about 5 minutes. Top the pizza with shredded lettuce, the reserved bacon and cheese, and the pico de gallo. Cut the pizza into 12 slices and garnish each slice with a dollop of sour cream and a slice of jalapeño.

Chapter 10

BACON IS MEAT CANDY

"I love bacon. My favorite thing is when meat and candy come together. So I like any kind of cured, sugary meat. My brother Neal likes to put a lot of sugar on bacon when he puts it in the oven, and that makes it very sweet. My favorite thing to do next would be to wrap it around chocolate. And then eat sugary bacon wrapped around like a chocolate Twix bar. Bacon makes everything a delight. Cannibalism becomes acceptable if you wrap a little bacon around the arm before you start chomping away."
—Conan O'Brien

INCLUDING BACON IN a dessert is not as crazy as it sounds. It's actually a really beautiful thing when done correctly. Thankfully, for their own sakes, people across the country are warming up to this idea and learning that sweet bacon isn't so scary after all. Usually it takes getting someone to sample a bacon-blessed dessert before they're willing to accept that it's no crazier than carrots in a cake. But the campaign to convince people to embrace the concept is far from complete.

BACON DESSERT: DON'T KNOCK IT UNTIL YOU'VE TRIED IT

Chef Greggory Hill (of course he'd put bacon in dessert!) knows the beauty of combining bacon with sweet flavors better than anyone else. His Bacon S'More is a chocolate soufflé with a slight but detectable taste of smoky bacon. The bacon is strong enough to give a kick to the moist chocolate treat—which is served with a side of vanilla ice cream—but not overwhelming or distracting. It is, in fact, totally complementary. When you're licking the plate clean, you will never again question the sanity of putting bacon in a dessert.

It seems that people's resistance to the idea of bacon in dessert generally has less to do with their own experience and more to do with their inability to accept the thought of meat in a dessert in general. Chef Hill believes it simply has to do with familiarity and comfort zones. "People think it's okay to do bacon for breakfast, lunch, or dinner, but if you put it into dessert, then they say, 'Oh, why are you doing that? That won't work!' Until they taste it. And then they get it." Chef Hill pushes the envelope when it comes to cooking bacon, and he is continually surprised by what people like and how hard it is to invent a dish they aren't willing to try. "I thought, for the longest time, it was going to be the bacon ice cream [that customers would have the most trouble with]. But people really like it. And it's not unusual anymore."

David Lebovitz is a pastry chef who received much of his training at Alice Waters's world-famous restaurant Chez Panisse in Berkeley, California. He has published several dessert books, including *The Perfect Scoop*, a guide to ice cream and frozen desserts.

David lives in Paris and publishes a blog, Living the Sweet Life in Paris. From his experience as a European resident, David has a different take on whether or not people are open to the idea of meat in dessert. "I think it's funny for Americans, perhaps, but other cultures have their meat-based desserts—mincemeat, for example—so it's not that weird. Unless you find mincemeat weird." He makes a good point, and assuming a certain segment of the world's population feels the same way, it's hard to believe that bacon in dessert isn't more commonplace.

In early 2008, David published an article on his Web site that featured a recipe for candied bacon ice cream. It became an instant hit with the online food-enthusiast community. The inspiration for it came from the idea of combining some of his favorite flavors into something unique yet simple. "I liked the idea of bacon and eggs and brown sugar together," says David (who doesn't?). "I knew of a molecular chef in England doing a riff on this but his recipe was hyper-complicated. So I wanted to make it simple, pare it down. And I like the idea of little nuggets in the ice cream, not a smooth, creamy emulsion." Anytime nuggets of bacon are involved, the outcome is always going to be good.

David experimented with a few different ways to candy the bacon, ranging from agave nectar to maple syrup to dark raw cane sugar. But in the end, the best result was with regular light brown sugar. He then mixed the crumbled caramelized bacon into a vanilla- and cinnamon-flavored ice cream.

David's ultimate taste test was to see what his butcher thought of the candied bacon ice cream. He didn't tell the butcher what was in the ice cream before he tasted it. But clearly it was a hit because the butcher polished off the sample and gave it a big thumbs up. A butcher is seemingly the kind of person who wouldn't be open to the idea of using meat in a blasphemous way, so his endorsement of bacon in a dessert should give more people the confidence to try their beloved bacon in new and different ways.

There are countless ways to experiment with bacon in a dessert. Bacon brownies, bacon chocolate chip cookies, and bacon pumpkin pie are just a few options that even the most inexperienced home cook could whip up with relative ease. Even if people you know have a hard time admitting that they like bacon in dessert, put it to a taste test and see what their stomachs have to say about it.

THE HUMAN-SWINE RELATIONSHIP

Numerous studies have been conducted regarding the close connection between humans and pigs. A few things we have in common:

- Pigs have very distinct individual personalities. Some are pleasant to be around; some are not.

- When raised in an open pasture, pigs like to romp and play games with one another as a way to pass the time.

- Pig organs can be used to save human lives—heart valve replacement is one such use that has been around for decades.

- Both humans and pigs have an affinity for trough-like environments. (Can you say "buffet line"?)

BACONCANDYLAND

In the last couple of years, several candy companies have caught on to the trend of combining bacon with sweet flavors. One of the top products in this category is the Vosges Haut-Chocolat candy bar called Mo's Bacon Bar. Mo's Bacon Bar combines the flavors and aromas of deep milk chocolate, alderwood-smoked bacon, and sea salt. The bacon bar has received some mixed reviews, but many people are also raving about it. If you've ever gone to the movies and dumped a bag of M&M's into your popcorn tub, then you'll understand the culinary phenomenon that makes the Mo's Bar so delicious. Beyond the bacon bar, Vosges takes a really unique approach to their high-end chocolate products. Almost all of their chocolate bars contain an unusual ingredient that has been inspired by an indigenous culture from around the world. Owner and chocolatier Katrina Markoff personally selects the ingredients used to produce their chocolate bars to create a sensory journey for her consumers. In addition to bacon, Vosges sells chocolate bars that contain ingredients such as red chiles (another appetizing combo), kalamata olives, curry, and wasabi. If you're ever in New York, Chicago, or Las Vegas, it's worth stopping by one of the Vosges boutiques for both the visual and taste experience. You can also order from Vosges over the Internet, and some of their products, including the Mo's Bacon Bar, are available in gourmet grocery stores in the United States. Bottom line: go find one wherever you can. You won't regret it.

Bacon peanut brittle is another bacon-infused treat that is incredibly delicious. To offer this product, The Grateful Palate partners with Tracey Dempsey, the pastry chef at a quirky upscale Southwestern-themed restaurant in Scottsdale, Arizona, called Cowboy Ciao. Your reaction to bacon peanut brittle will likely not be one of extreme like or dislike but rather surprise as to why no one had invented bacon brittle prior to this point in history. It just seems so natural. The bacon has a similar effect on the brittle as peanuts. The flavors blend together so well and so naturally that you could easily substitute the peanuts with bacon and there's a pretty good chance most people wouldn't even notice the difference. They would just know it's splendid.

Coco Rouge is a chocolatier based in Chicago that is also experimenting with bacon-blessed confections. Their bacon walnut toffee comes in bite-size pieces stored in a glass jar that you can easily keep in the kitchen cupboard and grab when you're in need of a quick fix for your sweet tooth. Or you could keep the jar on the coffee table so you can snack on the toffee while watching TV. Or you could keep a jar at your bedside so you can grab a handful of the delicious crunchy toffee when you wake up at 3:00 A.M. and need a little bite of something. Manage your snacking habits however you need to, but just know that Coco Rouge bacon walnut toffee is dangerously addictive.

Taking hardened bacon candy to the next level is a company called Lollyphile. This California-based purveyor of uniquely flavored lollipops introduced the Bacon Nation to the maple bacon lollipop in 2007. Using organic bacon and pure Vermont maple syrup, the folks at Lollyphile are boldly pushing the boundaries of using meat to manufacture candy. Their creation takes the best breakfast flavors and distills them down into a small piece of hard candy on a stick. The maple bacon lollipop has received some of the same criticism experienced by other bacon-based confectioners, but regardless of whether or not you like the candy, you really have to respect the ingenuity and bravado behind the invention.

Lollyphile founder Jason Lewis started his company with an absinthe-flavored lollipop as his first product. The maple bacon lollipop followed shortly thereafter: "I needed something not alcohol-based so that people would quit calling me at weird hours asking if my absinthe lollies would get them wasted (they won't), like I was a drug dealer. So I brainstormed: what do people really like, but that no one's ever seen in candy before? Oh, right—bacon. The maple bit just sort of followed suit." It was an instant hit.

Jason's favorite comment from a customer about his maple bacon lollipop? "Jesus got my letter!" Jason subsequently appended his Lollyphile marketing materials with this declaration of glee.

Now that the concept of bacon as candy is becoming more widely accepted, some chefs are taking their restaurant creations to a whole new level. One such chef is Sean Brock of McCrady's Restaurant in Charleston, South Carolina, who created bacon cotton candy.

Chef Brock's inspiration for bacon cotton candy came from a friend who shared a technique for making fat-based cotton candy. "Bacon was my first thought because it's my favorite thing in the world." The reaction from his customers has been nothing but positive. "People go nuts over it . . . we have served it to hundreds of people, people actually request it all the time." If only he could easily sell bacon cotton candy via mail order, then the world would be a better place.

Chef Brock has also experimented with bacon in other unusual ways. "We make a clear broth that tastes like bacon, which we can then whip into a foam or lots of other crazy stuff. I also like making bacon powder . . . it is stark white and tastes like really tasty smoked bacon." Just when you think you've seen it all in terms of bacon, someone like Chef Brock comes along and blows open the doors of the Bacon Nation.

You don't have to be a top chef to experiment with bacon in new and unusual ways. In an earlier chapter, bacon-wrapped hot dogs were discussed (with glee). But according to Greg, one of the readers of Bacon Unwrapped, one of the best bacon recipes he has ever tasted combines the savory flavors of a bacon-wrapped hot dog with the sweet and spicy flavors of raspberry and chipotle. According to Greg, "I was introduced to this wonderful delight at my local supermarket. They have a small kitchen area in the middle of the meat and cheese aisle where they promote various store products by cooking up fresh samples and handing out recipe cards. On that day I was drawn in by the sweet smell of bacon. The recipe is very simple. Just take your favorite hot dogs, wrap them with a strip of bacon (I use maple bacon), and fry them in a pan while drizzling a bottle of raspberry-chipotle sauce over them. I like to take the leftover bacon and fry it up with a little raspberry chipotle. Those flavors were meant to be together."

There is always going to be a segment of the population hesitant about using bacon in unusual ways such as dessert, regardless of how good these products might be. But those of us who are advocates of the Bacon Dessert Movement will continue our march forward.

BACON 'N' BOOZE

If you don't have much of a sweet tooth, there are lots of other unusual ways to use bacon that don't involve dessert. An increasingly popular trend at restaurants and bars is the use of bacon in cocktails. Booze and bacon. Bacon and booze. Both are addictive. Both make you feel happy. Both are a good reason to get out of bed in the morning. The two really have so much in common—it only makes sense to marry them in the form of a cocktail.

One of the more common booze-related uses for bacon is as a garnish for a Bloody Mary cocktail—also known as a Bacon Bloody. So while we're on this topic, let's take a tour of bacon bloodys across America.

At Tonic Restaurant in the Foggy Bottom neighborhood of Washington, DC, the bacon bloody is called Porky's Revenge, a house-made Bloody Mary with a crisp bacon swizzle stick. Indulge, but just be careful, though, because this refreshing cocktail might inspire you to go streaking through the nearby campus of George Washington University.

Moving farther west, the brunch menu at Sepia in Chicago offers a bacon Bloody Mary made with bacon-infused vodka and house-made Bloody Mary mix. The Sepia bacon bloody may not inspire you to go streaking, but it will make you want to extend brunch well into the afternoon.

According to a Bacon Unwrapped reader who goes by the user-name of sarstani, "Comet Cafe in Milwaukee, Wisconsin, has fabulous Bloody Marys with bacon in them next to the olives. I love going there for brunch on the weekends. They also have a free basket of bacon on Sunday evenings with any purchase of food. Bacon lovers flock from all over the city for that deliciousness." Being in the beer capital of the world, Comet Cafe also offers the option of having a Miller High Life chaser with your bacon bloody.

The Double Down Saloon—which has outlets in both New York City and Las Vegas—considers their bacon Bloody Mary to be part of a complete breakfast. And in 24/7 cities such as New York and Las Vegas, a bacon bloody breakfast is a meal that could occur any time of day. Just another benefit of being an American. And a bacon junkie.

At the annual Blue Ribbon Bacon Festival in Des Moines, bacon bloodys are one of many bacon concoctions served throughout the day. At this festival dedicated to The Best Meat Ever, you can eat and drink bacon to your heart's content (note: your heart also might appreciate a Lipitor chaser).

If you don't have bacon on hand, the guys who invented Bacon Salt have suggested using their flavored salt to make a bacon bloody instead of using the real thing—an idea that has the added benefit of being completely kosher.

Bacon as a garnish for booze just isn't enough for some bacon lovers, however. The art of directly infusing vodka with bacon is becoming a favorite hobby for some bacon lovers. For their second annual bacon eating contest, Atwood's Tavern in Cambridge, Massachusetts, created a bacon-infused vodka for BLT Bloody Marys that were garnished with lettuce and a cherry tomato. Sepia in Chicago also makes their own bacon-infused vodka for use in their bacon Bloody Marys. But you don't have to be a professional bartender to experiment with bacon-infused vodka. Several bloggers have experimented with it in the last couple of years and you can find their step-by-step instructions online so you don't have to reinvent the wheel.

Bacon-infused whiskey is another fun way to experiment with making your booze taste like bacon. Given that Jack Daniel's whiskey was born in the South, and the South is also a hotbed of bacon makin' activity, the two seem to go hand in hand. There are a handful of bartenders and bloggers currently working to create the perfect bacon whiskey. And where this is a will, there will most definitely be a way if bacon is involved.

Hard liquor isn't the only way to enjoy the flavor of bacon in your favorite libation. There is even a beer that claims to taste like bacon. Schlenkerla Brewery in Germany brews a rauchbier (smoke beer) with a distinctively smoky taste very reminiscent of bacon. This beer is not easy to find in the United States, but there are a few importers who sell the product if you're eager to give it a try. But be warned—this product is not for the faint of heart. It really, truly tastes like bacon in the form of a beer. The first couple of sips are a bit shocking, but once your palate gets used to the taste, it isn't quite as overwhelming. This author once took a few bottles to an Oktoberfest party. The host of the party appreciated the gesture, but then declared it to be one of the most disgusting things he has ever tasted. Whether it was because there weren't enough people at the party of Bavarian descent or because my openness to all things porcine has reached a new level of blind devotion, I was the only person to finish a bottle of rauchbier. This is one party favor idea that probably shouldn't be repeated.

THE STATE OF THE BACON NATION

Whether or not you think some of these unusual bacon combinations are delicious, the fact that people are coming up with them and a certain segment of the general public seems relatively open to trying them says a lot about the role bacon is playing in society today. The fact that bacon is not only being featured in some of the best restaurants in the country but that some restaurant patrons are visiting these restaurants specifically for that bacon speaks volumes about the way people view bacon. Bacon has evolved way, way, way beyond its initial role as a means of food preservation.

It is fascinating that bacon is experiencing such an increase in popularity at this point in time. Theories abound, but the most obvious reason why it's so popular is because it's The Best Meat Ever. On that note, here are a few additional thoughts to ponder.

First, the general public's interest level in food is at an all-time high thanks to the Food Network, the rise to prominence of celebrity chefs, and other food-related programming and media. People are paying more attention to the topic of food than ever before. They're cooking more at home and are more aware of the food they eat. Because of that, we're all becoming more aware of the numerous bacon options available to us beyond the major brands at the supermarket, and people are starting to branch out and try new—and in many cases, better—kinds of bacon.

Second, several of the more popular food celebrities (such as Anthony Bourdain, Paula Deen, and Emeril Lagasse) are big fans of all things pork-related, and all of them have a special place in their heart for bacon. It's doubtful that a day goes by on the Food Network without bacon being mentioned at least a couple of times. Because fans of these food celebrities respect what they have to say, they are going to naturally follow their lead when it comes to the foods they take an interest in, especially if that interest is in bacon.

Third, because of the increased visibility of bacon thanks to celebrity awareness, in the last few years there have been several prominent articles about the wonderful world of bacon in newspapers, magazines, and on popular food Web sites. The authors of these articles have covered bacon from numerous angles including the bacon blogosphere, Bacon of the Month clubs, quirky bacon-related products like bacon Band-Aids and bacon scarves, and chefs who use bacon prolifically.

Finally, several fast-food restaurants have recently added more bacon to their menu as a way to differentiate themselves from competitors. And the marketing of those products has resulted in some very creative advertising that puts bacon front and center, sometimes in very humorous and entertaining ways.

All of these factors combined together have led to an increase in bacon consumption in the United States over the last five years. Almost every independent bacon producer will acknowledge that their bacon sales have increased dramatically during that time period. The major brands have also experienced an increase in sales recently. To wrap it up, bacon is all the rage right now. And given that bacon is The Best Meat Ever, its popularity is unlikely to decline anytime soon.

CANDIED BACON ICE CREAM

This recipe comes from David Lebovitz, a chef and author currently living in Paris. The candied bacon nuggets perfectly complement the sweet vanilla ice cream. No other concoction better exemplifies the concept of bacon as meat candy.

MAKES ABOUT ¾ QUART

FOR THE CANDIED BACON

5 strips bacon
About 2 tablespoons light brown sugar

FOR THE ICE CREAM

3 tablespoons (⅜ stick) salted butter
¾ cup packed light or dark brown sugar (you can use either)
2¾ cups half-and-half
5 large egg yolks
2 teaspoons dark rum or whiskey
¼ teaspoon vanilla extract
¼ teaspoon ground cinnamon (optional)

1. To candy the bacon, preheat the oven to 400°F. Line a rimmed baking sheet with a silicone mat or aluminum foil, shiny side down. Sprinkle 1½ to 2 teaspoons brown sugar evenly over each strip of bacon, depending on length. Bake for 12 to 16 minutes. Midway during baking, flip the bacon strips over and drag them through the dark, syrupy liquid that's collected on the baking sheet. Continue to bake until as dark as mahogany. Remove from the oven and cool the strips on a wire rack. Once crisp and cool, chop the bacon into little pieces, about the size of grains of rice.

(The bacon bits can be stored in an airtight container and chilled in the refrigerator for a day or so before use, or stored in the freezer a few weeks ahead.)

2. To make the ice cream, melt the butter in a heavy, medium saucepan over low heat. Stir in the brown sugar and half of the half-and-half. Pour the remaining half-and-half into a bowl (preferably metal) set in an ice bath and set a mesh strainer over the top. Cook the sugar-cream mixture, stirring occasionally, just until the sugar has dissolved completely. Do not boil.

3. In a separate bowl, stir together the egg yolks, then gradually add some of the warm sugar-cream mixture to them, whisking the yolks constantly as you pour. Pour the mixture back into the saucepan. Cook over low to moderate heat, constantly stirring and scraping the bottom with a heatproof spatula, until the custard thickens enough to coat the spatula.

4. Strain the custard into the bowl of half-and-half. Stir until cool. Stir in the liquor, vanilla, and cinnamon, if using. Refrigerate the mixture.

5. Once thoroughly chilled, freeze in your ice cream maker according to the manufacturer's instructions. Add the bacon bits during the last moment of churning, or stir them in when you remove the ice cream from the machine.

BACON BROWNIES

To make bacon brownies, the author modified a brownie recipe she once made for a 4-H county fair project twenty-five years ago. Don't use an overwhelming amount of bacon—use just enough to give the brownies a hint of the smoky bacon flavor, which complements the chocolate quite nicely.

MAKES ONE 13 X 9-INCH PAN OF BROWNIES

½ pound (2 sticks) margarine
½ cup unsweetened cocoa powder
2 cups sugar
4 large eggs
1½ cups all-purpose flour
Pinch of salt
4 strips bacon, cooked until crispy and finely chopped

Preheat the oven to 350°F. Grease a 13 x 9-inch baking pan. Melt the margarine in the microwave. Stir in the cocoa. In a separate large bowl, beat together the sugar and eggs. Add the flour and salt and mix well. Add the cocoa mixture and bacon and stir well. Pour the batter into the prepared pan. Bake for 30 to 35 minutes, until you can insert a toothpick into the center of the brownies and it comes out clean. This is best served warm, even better with a scoop of ice cream.

BACON, GRILLED CHEESE, AND
APPLE SANDWICH

"Bacon and apples? Seriously?" Understandably, you may be skeptical. But you're gonna have to trust Brenda Beaman of Williamson Kenwood and Rocco Loosbrock of Coastal Vineyards on this one. You'll never look at apples the same way again after eating them on this cheesy bacon-blessed sandwich. It's sweet, it's bacony, it's a little like dessert and a lot like lunch (you might want to experiment with an apple cinnamon–flavored bacon for this particular bacon adventure). Enjoy.

SERVES 4

12 slices bacon
2 Pink Lady apples (or whatever favorite kind of
　　apple you have easy access to)
½ pound sharp Cheddar cheese
Nonstick cooking spray
8 slices bread

1. Cook the bacon slices to your desired doneness. Remove the bacon and place it on a paper towel–lined plate.
2. While the bacon is cooking, slice the apples into quarters and remove the cores. Slice the apples into ⅛-inch-thick slices and set aside. Slice the cheese into ⅛-inch slices and set aside.
3. Heat a large skillet over medium heat and spray with nonstick cooking spray. Place one slice of bread in the skillet and layer with one quarter of the cheese, slices from half of an apple, and 3 whole slices of bacon. Top with a second slice of bread. Repeat with remaining ingredients.

4. When the first side has developed a golden brown crust, carefully flip the sandwich. Remove the sandwich from the skillet when the second side is also golden brown. Scarf it down immediately!

TODD GRAY'S BBQ SAUCE

To find bacon in a BBQ sauce isn't all that uncommon. However, what makes this recipe interesting is the use of Coca-Cola to give the sauce its sweet flavor. Once again, sugar and bacon proves to be an unstoppable duo. You'll want to spread this BBQ sauce all over any kind of grilled meat you can get your hands on. You might get a little crazy and smear it on the brownies featured in this section. Who knows? This recipe comes to us courtesy of Todd Gray, Executive Chef of Equinox Restaurant in Washington, DC.

MAKES 4 TO 5 CUPS

2 cups diced applewood-smoked bacon (about 6–8 strips)
1 small onion, preferably Vidalia, cut into large dice
1 tablespoon ground sumac (available at Middle Eastern stores)
1 tablespoon ground chipotle chile
1½ teaspoons red pepper flakes
3 cups apple cider vinegar
2 cups Coca-Cola
2 cups ketchup
Salt and pepper

1. Place a medium saucepan over medium-high heat. Add the bacon and cook, stirring occasionally, until it starts to give up its fat. Add the onion, sumac, chipotle, and red pepper flakes. Lower the heat

to medium and cook for 5 to 8 minutes, stirring occasionally, until the bacon and onion are golden brown.

2. Add the apple cider vinegar and stir to dislodge any browned bits on the bottom of the pan. Simmer until reduced by two thirds.

3. Add the Coca-Cola and simmer until reduced by half.

4. Add the ketchup and simmer for 4 minutes. Remove from the heat.

5. When the sauce has cooled slightly, puree in a blender. Pass through a fine-mesh strainer into a bowl or storage container. Season to taste with salt and pepper.

RESOURCES

THOSE WHO MAKE BACON

Aidells
www.aidells.com

Broadbent Hams
257 Mary Blue Road
Kuttawa, KY 42055
(800) 841-2202
www.broadbenthams.com

Burgers' Smokehouse
32819 Highway 97
California, MO 65018
(800) 345-5185
www.smokehouse.com

Danish Bacon
www.dbmc.co.uk

Father's Country Hams
P.O. Box 99
Bremen, KY 42325
(877) 525-4267
www.fatherscountryhams.com

Flying Pigs Farm
246 Sutherland Road
Shushan, NY 12873
(518) 854-3844
www.flyingpigsfarm.com

Hormel
www.hormel.com

La Quercia
400 Hakes Drive
Norwalk, IA 50211
(515) 981-1625
www.laquercia.us

LightLife (Smart Bacon)
www.lightlife.com

Newsom's Aged Kentucky
Country Hams
208 East Main Street
Princeton, KY 42445
(270) 365-2482
www.newsomscountryham.com

Niman Ranch
(888) 206-3327
www.nimanranch.com

Nueske's Applewood Smoked Meats
Rural Route #2, P.O. Box D
Wittenberg, WI 54499
(800) 392-2266
www.nueskes.com

Oscar Mayer
brands.kraftfoods.com/oscarmayer

The Pork Shop
3359 East Combs Road
Queen Creek, AZ 85240
(480) 987-0101

Scott Country Hams
1301 Scott Road
Greenville, KY 42345
(800) 318-1353
www.scotthams.com

Smithfield Foods
www.smithfield.com

Swiss Meat & Sausage Co.
2056 South Highway 19
Hermann, MO 65041
(800) 793-SWISS
www.swissmeats.com

Thielen's Meat Market
310 Main Street North
Pierz, MN 56364
(320) 468-6616

THOSE WHO DISTRIBUTE BACON

Coastal Vineyards
207 West Lost Angeles Avenue, #346
Moorpark, CA 93021
(877) 21-BACON
www.cvwine.com

D'Artagnan
(800) 327-8246
www.dartagnan.com

The Grateful Palate
(888) 472-5283
www.gratefulpalate.com

Zingerman's
422 Detroit Street
Ann Arbor, MI 48104
(888) 636-8162
www.zingermans.com

THOSE WHO WRITE ABOUT BACON

Bacon Salt Blog
www.baconsaltblog.com

The Bacon Show
baconshow.blogspot.com

Bacontarian
www.bacontarian.com

Bacon Today
www.bacontoday.com

Bacon Unwrapped
www.baconunwrapped.com

David Lebovitz
www.davidlebovitz.com

Fergus Henderson
www.stjohnrestaurant.co.uk

I ❤ Bacon
www.iheartbacon.com

International Bacon Day
internationalbaconday.blogspot.com

John Martin Taylor
www.hoppinjohns.com

Lords of Bacon
www.lordsofbacon.com

Lounge of Tomorrow
www.loungeoftomorrow.com

Mad Meat Genius
www.madmeatgenius.com

Michael Ruhlman
blog.ruhlman.com

Mr. Baconpants
www.mrbaconpants.com

Peter Kaminsky
Author of *Pig Perfect: Encounters with Remarkable Swine and Some Great Ways to Cook Them* (Hyperion, 2005), a must-read for any pork enthusiast

Royal Bacon Society
www.royalbaconsociety.com

Sarah Katherine Lewis
www.sexandbacon.com

Sara Perry
www.saraperry.com

Skulls and Bacon
skullsandbacon.blogspot.com

THOSE RESTAURANTS THAT DO BACON PROUD

ARIZONA

Cowboy Ciao
7133 East Stetson Drive
Scottsdale, AZ 85251
(480) WINE-111
www.cowboyciao.com

Matt's Big Breakfast
801 North 1st Street
Phoenix, AZ 85004
(602) 254-1074
www.mattsbigbreakfast.com

Richardson's
1582 East Bethany Home Road
Phoenix, AZ 85014
(602) 265-5886
www.burningembersphoenix.com

CALIFORNIA

Godspeed Café
5532 San Pablo
Oakland, CA 94608
(510) 547-1313
www.godspeed.bz

Pink's Hot Dogs
709 North La Brea Boulevard
Los Angeles, CA 90038
(323) 931-4223
www.pinkshollywood.com

DISTRICT OF COLUMBIA

Ben's Chili Bowl
1213 U Street NE
Washington, DC 20009
(202) 667-0909
www.benschilibowl.com

BLT Steak
1625 Eye Street NW
Washington, DC 20006
(202) 689-8999
www.bltsteak.com

Equinox Restaurant
818 Connecticut Avenue NW
Washington, DC 20006
(202) 331-8118
www.equinoxrestaurant.com

Mio Restaurant
1110 Vermont Avenue NW
Washington, DC 20005
(202) 955-0075
www.miorestaurant.com

Rock Creek Restaurant
5300 Wisconsin Avenue, NW
Washington, DC 20015
(202) 966-7625
www.rockcreekrestaurant.com

Tonic Restaurant
2036 G Street NW
Washington, DC 20036
(202) 296-0021
www.tonicrestaurant.com

IDAHO

Brick 29
320 11th Avenue South
Nampa, ID 83651
(208) 468-0029
www.brick29.com

ILLINOIS

Alinea Restaurant
1723 North Halstead
Chicago, IL 60614
(312) 867-0110
www.alinea-restaurant.com

Sepia Restaurant
123 North Jefferson Street
Chicago, IL 60661
(312) 441-1920
www.sepiachicago.com

Whiskey Road
1935 North Damen Avenue
Chicago, IL 60647
(773) 315-2540
www.whiskeyroadchicago.com

IOWA

High Life Lounge
200 S.W. 2nd Street
Des Moines, IA 50309
(515) 280-1965
www.thehighlifelounge.com

KENTUCKY

The Brown Hotel
335 West Broadway
Louisville, KY 40202
(502) 583-1234
www.brownhotel.com

Ramsey's Diner
496 East High Street
Lexington, KY 40507
(859) 259-2708
www.ramseysdiners.com

MASSACHUSETTS

Atwood's Tavern
877 Cambridge Street
Cambridge, MA 02141
(617) 864-2792
www.atwoodstavern.com

MINNESOTA

Manny's Steakhouse
821 Marquette Avenue South
Minneapolis, MN 55402
(612) 215-3700
www.mannyssteakhouse.com

Psycho Suzi's Motor Lounge
2519 Marshall Street NE
Minneapolis, MN 55418
(612) 788-9069
www.psychosuzis.com

The Triple Rock Social Club
629 Cedar Avenue
Minneapolis, MN 55454
(612) 333-7499
www.triplerocksocialclub.com

NEVADA

CatHouse (Luxor Hotel and Casino)
3900 Las Vegas Boulevard South
Las Vegas, NV 89229
(877) 386-4658
www.luxor.com/nightlife/cathouse.
aspx

Double Down Saloon
4640 Paradise Road
Las Vegas, NV 89169
(702) 791-5775
www.doubledownsaloon.com

NEW YORK

Crif Dogs (Manhattan)
113 St. Marks Place
New York, NY 10009
(212) 614-2728

Peter Luger Steakhouse
178 Broadway
Brooklyn, NY 11211
(718) 387-7400
www.peterluger.com

OHIO

Lola
2058 E. 4th Street
Cleveland, OH 44115
(216) 621-5652
www.lolabistro.com

Lolita
900 Literary Road
Tremont, OH 44113
(216) 771-5652
www.lolabistro.com

OREGON

Voodoo Doughnuts
22 S.W. Third Avenue
Portland, OR 97204
(503) 241-4704
www.voodoodoughnut.com

PENNSYLVANIA

Fatheads
1805 East Carson Street
Pittsburgh, PA 15203
(412) 431-7433
www.fatheads.com

Harris Grill
5747 Ellsworth Avenue
Pittsburgh, PA 15232
(412) 362-5273
www.harrisgrill.com

SOUTH CAROLINA

McCrady's Restaurant
2 Unity Alley
Charleston, SC 29401
(843) 577-0025
www.mccradysrestaurant.com

VIRGINIA

Bob & Edith's Diner
2310 Columbia Pike
Arlington, VA 22204
(703) 920-6103

EatBar and Tallula
2761 Washington Boulevard
Arlington, VA 22201
(703) 778-9951
www.tallularestaurant.com

WISCONSIN

Comet Cafe
1947 North Farwell Avenue
Milwaukee, WI 53202
(414) 273-7677
www.thecometcafe.com

THOSE WHO SERVE BACON TO THE MASSES

Applebee's
www.applebees.com

A&W Restaurants
www.awrestaurants.com

Bojangles'
www.bojangles.com

Chili's Grill and Bar
www.chilis.com

Cracker Barrel Old Country Store
and Restaurant
www.crackerbarrel.com

Denny's
www.dennys.com

Five Guys Burgers and Fries
www.fiveguys.com

McDonald's
www.mcdonalds.com

The Original Pancake House
www.originalpancakehouse.com

Red Robin
www.redrobin.com

Sonic Drive-In
www.sonicdrivein.com

Waffle House
www.wafflehouse.com

Wendy's
www.wendys.com

THOSE WHO EXPRESS LOVE OF BACON IN UNIQUE WAYS

Accoutrements
www.accoutrements.com
(wholesale only)

Archie McPhee
www.mcphee.com

Bacon Salt
www.baconsalt.com

Baconwrapt Scarves
www.baconwrapt.com

Coco Rouge
www.cocorouge.com

Flavor Spray
www.flavor-spray.com

Lollyphile
www.lollyphile.com

Sappy Moose Tree
www.sappymoosetree.com

Schlenkerla Brewery
www.schlenkerla.de/indexe.html

Shopsin's General Store
www.shopsinsgeneralstore.com

Vosges Haut-Chocolat
www.vosgeschocolate.com

THOSE WHO TEACH US ABOUT BACON

National Pork Board
www.pork.org

National Pork Producers Council
www.nppc.org

National Sustainable Agriculture
Information Service
attra.ncat.org

Slow Food USA
www.slowfoodusa.org

Southern Foodways Alliance
www.southernfoodways.com

THOSE WHO CELEBRATE BACON

Bacon and Bean Days
Augusta, WI
www.augustawi.com

Living History Farms
11121 Hickman Road
Urbandale, IA 50322
(515) 278-5286
www.lhf.org

Preble County Pork Festival
Preble County Fairgrounds
722 South Franklin Street
Eaton, OH 45320
www.porkfestival.org

Tipton County Pork Festival
Tipton, IN 46072
(765) 675-2342
www.tiptoncountyporkfestival.com

Virginia Pork Festival
425 South Main Street
Emporia, VA 23847
800-4-VA-PORK
www.vaporkfestival.com

World Pork Expo
Iowa State Fairgrounds
E. 30th Street and E. University
    Avenue
Des Moines, IA 50317
www.worldpork.org

Gailtaler Speckfest
Hermagor, Austria
www.gailtalerspeck.at

INDEX